"Dr. Shenkman provides a proven and comprehensive plan to keep you at your peak fitness and, ultimately, put herself out of work! Her long years as a doctor and athlete add to the importance of this work. Share it widely with your friends and loved ones as I will."

—Joel Kahn, MD, FACC, Author of *The Plant-Based Solution*

"If you don't want to be another victim of the obesity and heart disease epidemic, then read this eye-opening, inspiring, and very practical book by Dr. Shenkman. You will quickly discover that we have so much more control over our health and destiny than we are led to believe once we have the right knowledge and tools. Reading this book will give you precisely what you need to turn your life and health around now and never look back—the comprehensive information in this book that Dr. Shenkman shares can literally add both years to your life and life to your years!"

**—Steven Lawenda, MD, Family Medicine
and Lifestyle Medicine**

"There's a movement afoot in healthcare to address cardiovascular disease at the root: our diets. And there's no one better equipped to speak out about the deleterious effects of the standard American diet (appropriately abbreviated to SAD) than a cardiologist like Dr. Heather Shenkman. The evidence for the efficacy of dietary changes in the prevention and treatment of many diseases is clear, and now is the time to put plant-based diets on the forefront. This book not only clearly explains the case for eating more plant foods, but shows you how to do it. *The Vegan Heart Doctor's Guide* is a gift to the world that can literally save lives!"

—Matt Ruscigno, MPH, RD, Chief Nutrition Officer at Nutrinic

"Diet is now the number-one cause of early death and disability in the United States. The beautiful message from that is we have much control over our health destiny based on what we put on the end of our fork. Dr. Shenkman provides a sound starting point with tools to empower patients to help reduce, and even prevent, symptoms and adverse health outcomes associated with cardiovascular disease."

—Julieanna Hever, MS, RD, CPT, Author of the *Plant-Based Nutrition Idiot's Guide* and *The Vegiterranean Diet*

"This book contains the words of a woman who has 'done the work.' Dr. Shenkman takes your hand and guides you through dramatic lifestyle changes in a completely digestible manner. Not one person who reads and follows the simple guidelines of this book will lack health ever again. From understanding matters of the heart from a clinical standpoint to choosing an appropriate exercise regime and adopting healthy eating habits, there is no stone left unturned. You will finish this book as a well-educated, motivated participant in your life, ready to take charge and live the life you were always meant to live."

—Jess Gumkowski, Co-Founder of YogiTriathlete, Endurance Athlete, Podcast Host, Vegan Lifestyle Coach and Educator, and Author of *YogiTriathlete Cookbook: High-Vibe Recipes for the Athlete Appetite*

"Dr. Shenkman has done it! Heed the words in this book as you would passages in the Bible; they are that important. I should know. I became the first male in my family in three generations to reach the age of fifty and finally break free from our heart disease curse, and it is all thanks to Dr. Shenkman. Bravo!"

—Derek Gray, Certified Personal Trainer, Author of *When We Were Five* and *How to Stop Being Lazy and Start Living Healthy*

"Dr. Shenkman personally provided me with life-changing information and support after the discovery of my nearly fatal cardiovascular disease. With a small dose of self-discipline, this book provides all the information you'll need to put you on a path to a healthier lifestyle and improved quality of life!"

—Michael Richardson

THE VEGAN
HEART DOCTOR'S GUIDE
to Reversing Heart Disease, Losing Weight,
and Reclaiming Your Life

HEATHER SHENKMAN, MD, FACC

FOREWORD BY NEAL D. BARNARD, MD, FACC

Published by:
Tofu Triathlete Publishing
18663 Ventura Blvd., Suite 202
Tarzana, CA 91356
Phone: 818-938-9505
Fax: 818-938-9513
Email: dr@drheathershenkman.com
www.drheathershenkman.com

ISBN: 978-0-999-76761-0

Library of Congress Control Number: 2017919578

Printed in the United States of America

I dedicate this book to my parents, Gail and Jack Shenkman, who have always encouraged me to pursue medicine and follow my dreams. I also dedicate this book to my inspiring patients, who always impress me with their willingness to learn and their ability to adapt and improve their lifestyles to achieve better health.

Table of Contents

FOREWORD

The world of medicine changed in 1990. That was the year that Dr. Dean Ornish, a young Harvard-trained physician, set out to see whether heart disease could be not only prevented, but *reversed.* Up until that point, most doctors relied on drugs and surgery to treat heart problems, and often they hoped only to slow the progression of the disease, rather than truly restore their patients' health.

Dr. Ornish wanted to go further. He invited patients in the San Francisco Bay area to join a research study. He did not use cholesterol-lowering drugs, angioplasty, or bypass surgery. Instead he used a simple program of a low-fat vegetarian diet, easy exercise (a half-hour daily walk), stress management techniques, and smoking cessation. A control group followed their regular doctors' advice, which typically meant a chicken-and-fish diet, along with cholesterol-lowering drugs.

After a year, the participants were evaluated. In the vegetarian group, the average person's cholesterol had dropped 24 percent, which was great. LDL ("bad") cholesterol had dropped a whopping 37 percent. When they stood on the scale, the average person had lost 22 pounds, which certainly got their attention. But the most important result was when each patient had an angiogram, a special X-ray that measures artery blockages. The results were compared to the same test done at the beginning of the study, and the findings made medical history. The arteries had stopped narrowing. Instead, they had begun to reopen so much that the tests showed a measurable difference in 82 percent of the participants in the first year. All this from a simple regimen of vegetarian foods, easy exercise, stress management, and no smoking.

When the results appeared, I called Dr. Ornish. I said that doctors would believe that the regimen worked, but they would also imagine that no one could ever follow what seemed like a very strict regimen. So, he invited me to come to San Francisco and put that question to the test. I took him up on the offer and interviewed all the participants. I asked them to rate how well they liked the food, how much effort the diet required to prepare it, how their families reacted, whether they would prefer the diet or prescription medications, and whether they planned to stick with it in the future. It turned out that the vegetarian group did grumble a bit. They said it took about six weeks to really get 100 percent comfortable with it. But they also found that their tastes had changed and that they liked the new way of eating. More importantly, their chest pain was gone, they had lost weight effortlessly, and they felt better than they had in years. Stop the diet? No way, they said.

A bigger surprise was the control group. They grumbled, too, saying that their diet was boring, consisting of just chicken and fish and chicken and fish and chicken and fish, night after night. All the pleasures of life were gone, and they had nothing to show for it. They still had chest pain, and they still had worsening heart disease.

One of the interviews really stood out in my mind. One of the men in the vegetarian group was palpably angry. I asked him what the matter was. He said that the research study had been a life-changing experience and that the diet had very likely saved his life. But he was very troubled—and frankly furious—that no doctor had ever told him about this before. They had been ready to write prescription after prescription, do risky heart surgery, and charge him tens of thousands of dollars, and, until he met Dr. Ornish, not a single one had ever thought to suggest that he could improve his health on his own, with simple lifestyle changes. "Too many doctors have projected their own values onto other people who don't share them," he said.

Five years later, Dr. Ornish published his long-term research results in the *Journal of the American Medical Association*, showing that the diet program dramatically cut the likelihood of ever having a heart attack, being hospitalized needing heart surgery, or dying from heart problems.

At the Cleveland Clinic, Dr. Caldwell Esselstyn showed that this sort of healthful diet change essentially obliterates heart disease. And by now, many people have started to put this approach to work for themselves.

In our research at the Physicians Committee for Responsible Medicine, we have found that a similar diet adjustment is also great for people who don't have heart problems. It tackles weight problems easily, without calorie counting or portion limits. It improves high blood pressure and diabetes, and sometimes even makes these conditions go away entirely. Joint pains, migraines, and other health problems often improve dramatically.

Many other researchers have explored the power of diet changes. Together, we have shown that a healthful menu built from vegetables, fruits, grains, and beans is good, not just for people with health problems, but for everyone. It turns out to be surprisingly easy, and the foods are very likely more varied and delicious than what you're eating now.

This book will help you to put the power of foods and a healthful lifestyle to work in your own life. Dr. Heather Shenkman's experience and wisdom will explain what you need to know and show you how to get started.

Dr. Shenkman knows what she is talking about. She is not just a highly trained physician and cardiologist. As you will see, she once followed a not-so-healthful diet herself, and she has made the same changes that you are about to jump into. She will guide you every step of the way. You will find that it is surprisingly easy and the payoff is enormous. Soon, you will see what it will do for you.

I hope you enjoy the new path you're on, and that you will share your success with others.

Neal D. Barnard, MD, FACC
Adjunct Associate Professor of Medicine, George Washington University School of Medicine
President, Physicians Committee for Responsible Medicine
Washington, DC

PREFACE

What I love most about being a cardiologist is that I can make a difference in the world by saving a life. I am able to open the blocked artery of a sick person in the throes of a heart attack and give them a second chance. Or, I can share with my patients proven healing methods to prevent another heart attack from happening in the future, or possibly even prevent a heart attack in the first place.

While there are many things that I can do to help people feel better and live longer, many people do not realize that their own actions are the key to their success as cardiac patients. From understanding what heart disease is to knowing how and why to take their medications and recognizing the important role of a healthy diet and lifestyle, patients themselves have much power to control their own destiny. Perhaps you are one of these patients, longing to take control of your cardiac health but unsure of what to do and where to start. If so, I encourage you to read this book thoroughly and recognize your own healing potential. You really do have the power to impact your own health.

With this book, I have put into words all that I want to convey to my patients, or any patients who are concerned about their heart health. I want to motivate them to make positive changes to their diet and exercise habits, to move forward, and to be as healthy as possible. It is my hope that as you read these pages you will feel empowered, hopeful, and emboldened to defeat heart disease and give yourself a second chance at a better life.

ACKNOWLEDGMENTS

I thank those who made this book possible. Most importantly, I'd like to say thank you to my parents, Gail and Jack Shenkman, for their never-ending support throughout my life. To the physicians I've had the honor to work with, from medical school, through residency and fellowship, to my 10 years in private practice: Thank you for inspiring me throughout my career. To my patients, who show me that it's never too late to make positive lifestyle changes. Thank you to Dottie DeHart, Eve Campbell, and the entire team at DeHart & Company Public Relations for all their hard work on this book. And my deepest thanks to Dr. Caldwell Esselstyn and Dr. Dean Ornish for their groundbreaking research that demonstrates the benefits of a plant-based diet.

INTRODUCTION

Paul, a patient of mine, never expected that he would have a heart attack. However, at only 44, he developed an unusual chest pain. He went to the emergency room, and much to his surprise, was told that he was in fact having a heart attack—a bad one.

An ambulance transfer later, he was in the cardiac catheterization laboratory undergoing angioplasty of his left anterior descending coronary artery—in other words, the "widow-maker" artery. This procedure likely saved his life. Another narrowed artery was noted on his angiogram pictures, and he was told he would likely need a second procedure to open that artery at a later date.

His doctors put him on the appropriate medications and discharged him from the hospital just a few days later. Motivated by the desire to avoid any further heart procedures, Paul read about the power of plant-based diets to reverse even the most severe heart disease. He decided right then to adopt a plant-based diet and immediately began eating exclusively vegan, whole-food, plant-based fare, with no nuts, oils, or avocado. He also began exercising more, by running and hiking the trails near his home five mornings per week.

As directed, he returned to his cardiologist for a stress test, to assess the significance of the damage to the remaining abnormal artery. As it turned out, the stress test for that portion of the heart was completely normal, and he never required the second angioplasty that he was told he would need.

Over two years after his heart attack, he has continued to feel well. He enjoys his healthy diet and says that he does not find it hard to follow. He prepares meals with whole grains, vegetables, and satisfying proteins like lentils, beans, and tofu. His greatest challenge is when he travels for work and has to rely on restaurant food for his meals. But he finds that restaurants always accommodate his requests for plant-based meals if there is nothing specifically vegan on the menu and often relies on eating salads while traveling.

Paul was lucky to receive lifesaving medical intervention when he needed it, but the bigger victory is that he chose to make the lifestyle changes he so desperately needed. Given his overwhelming success on a plant-based diet, Paul is now trying to open the eyes of his family, particularly his father, who also had a heart attack more than 20 years ago. He is a great example of a patient who took charge of his health and is now reaping the rewards.

What if I told you that there is no reason why you should ever have another heart attack, require another stent, or suffer another cardiac event? That with the right medications, lifestyle, and diet you could have many healthy, happy, quality years ahead of you? I am not sure you would believe me if I told you these things. And the widespread presence of heart disease in America is the reason.

Too many people in this country, unfortunately, have suffered the harsh realities associated with heart attacks, stents, and bypass surgeries. In fact, one in every three deaths in the United States is attributable to cardiovascular disease.[1] One might think that the threat of a disease with such an enormous scope and impact would inspire people to work hard, overcome the odds, and improve their chances of staying healthy. But the truth is, in this terrifying battle, heart disease is winning.

And sadly, it's not really that surprising given the lifestyle of many Americans today. We live in a culture of overextended schedules and long work hours at stressful jobs, with little room left for relaxing, having fun with family and friends, or getting some much-needed fresh air and exercise. All of this stress is highly detrimental to our bodies and souls. And don't forget that despite the explicit warnings about the dangers of smoking and excessive alcohol consumption, many people throw caution to the wind and continue to smoke and drink with abandon. All of these factors have created the perfect storm in terms of heart disease.

Then, too, there's the giant conundrum over food in this country and the problems it has unleashed on society. The standard American diet undermines your heart at every turn and contributes to the current obesity crisis. Consider the abundance of cheaply made, fatty, salty, and sugary "fast food" that we have instant access to, whether from a drive-thru or on the shelves at the market. And while healthy whole food ingredients *are* available, they take a bit more time to prepare, and people are often too exhausted (in part because of their poor diets) to make a real effort to intentionally choose and prepare the meals they eat.

I hear this line of logic from my patients regularly. Instead of preparing healthy meals, they choose what is available fast and now: instant, meat-heavy, dairy-rich, super-processed dinners. Is it any wonder that our hearts are struggling to keep up with this unsustainable lifestyle?

And our lifestyles aren't the only problem. Doctors today are often very rushed, as they usually have a full roster of patients needing care. Getting the time you need from your doctor to learn about your heart condition can be difficult, and sometimes it can even be tough to get a timely appointment in the first place. And when you do see your doctor, she may not make the time to ask you about your lifestyle, nor to counsel you on optimal diet and exercise.

One reason this happens is because our healthcare system here in America is not adequately set up to encourage healthy lifestyles and prevention. Rather, it is built to pay for *treatment*, usually in the form of surgeries and prescriptions, after someone becomes sick—and the medical community is truly excellent in this aspect of care. However, we need to go further to educate patients on *preventing* illness, namely heart disease, in the first place. Though the Affordable Care Act is taking strides to respond to this systemic problem, we still have a long way to go.

Thanks to all of these factors, many, if not most, people feel hopeless and helpless when confronted with their heart health. They often feel doomed by their own genetics, which were first manifested by close family members who may have already succumbed to heart disease, destined to wait for the next heart attack, or for the next coronary artery stent to need to be placed, helplessly believing that their time on earth is limited, feeling that they have no recourse beyond submitting to their fate. And so they continue to make the same diet and lifestyle choices they have always made and wait for nature to take its course.

I know I have painted you a bleak picture here. But wouldn't you be surprised—thrilled even—if you learned that there is no reason why you should ever suffer another cardiac event? That, by working with your doctor, and taking positive steps to improve your lifestyle, you could reset your health and have many quality years ahead of you? I have some good news: You *can* say goodbye to heart disease forever. You can change your present, let go of your history, and change the course of your future.

I chose a career in cardiology because I knew it was a field where I could help people. I spent years in training to perform procedures to evaluate the heart, the ultrasounds and nuclear scans, and the invasive procedures to seemingly work magic to open blocked arteries. I am skilled to choose and prescribe medications to control blood pressure, lower cholesterol, and strengthen the heart.

However, even with these great advances in technology and research, heart disease is still a killer. How can that be the case? Again, it is our lifestyle that is holding us back. Our sedentary ways, fast food, animal products, junk food, alcohol, smoking, and the stress of our daily lives make the battle against heart disease all that more challenging. But the fact that this country has "normalized" the conditions that manifest heart disease is no reason to stand idly by and allow it to claim the lives of so many. At one time, heart attacks were rare, and I believe that with some effort and know-how, we can wipe heart disease off the map and enjoy excellent health.

I wrote this book to serve as a wake-up call to those at risk for and suffering from heart disease. I want to shake America from its complacency and tell everyone that their feelings of helplessness are untrue. We cannot accept that it is normal to have a heart attack. Heart attacks are not "normal," and heart disease, though terrible and pervasive, is not an unstoppable foe. Heart disease *can* be prevented and reversed. I fully believe that with the right care, there is no need to have a heart attack. With the right medications, lifestyle, and food choices, we can live longer, and more importantly, we can live better.

This book is for anyone who is concerned about his or her heart health. I hope to provide you the motivation and guidance to live a long, healthy, and happy life, free of heart disease. And, if you have had heart disease, I hope to help you to live for many years to come, free of any further heart problems or need for any type of heart procedures.

My goal is not to scare you. My goal is to get you to take action and to change your life. Maybe you've had a heart attack or have stents. Or maybe you've been fortunate thus far and have a healthy heart and hope to keep it that way. I want your heart to be as healthy as possible. Regardless of your current health, you can take action to not only live longer but live better. After all, none of us is perfect; we can all make changes to be even healthier than we are today.

I believe in conquering heart disease in an unconventional way and as naturally as possible. While my work as an interventional cardiologist is certainly valuable—as I am able to help save lives in the event of acute heart-related emergencies—my philosophy involves a more holistic approach to achieving wellness that can be implemented every day.

First, I strongly advocate adopting a plant-based diet and will later share the steps to undertaking this seemingly drastic change with ease. Research shows that a plant-based diet is not only healthy for you in general, but can actually reverse the effects of heart disease, reduce your risk of many other illnesses including diabetes and several kinds of cancer, and help you to live longer. And because you have complete control over your dietary choices, it stands to reason that making intelligent food choices is one of the simplest ways to achieve and maintain good health. In this book I will also cite hard evidence that verifies just how powerful and transformative a plant-based diet really is.

A second health factor entirely under your control is how much you exercise. You don't have to become a triathlete to glean the benefits of fitness. Even a simple walking routine can create a dramatic impact on your health. Later I will show you how to incorporate a manageable fitness routine into your life—and yes, how to have fun along the way.

I have dedicated my life to the pursuit of wellness, and I take pride in being able to help others do the same in the doctor's office, on the cath lab table, and beyond. I want to educate you and give you the tools to be as healthy and happy as possible. Read on and you will learn what heart disease is and what *you* can do to optimize your heart health, from taking the proper prescriptions to eating the right foods to getting the exercise your heart needs.

Heart Disease: A Formidable Killer

How Being a Cardiologist Has Shaped My "Good Health" Philosophy

By trade, I am an interventional cardiologist, trained to implant coronary stents in blocked arteries and to open the arteries of patients suffering heart attacks and save their lives. Yet I don't think of myself solely as a technician. While I enjoy the challenge of a complex angioplasty, and the satisfaction of helping someone with my invasive technical skills, my greatest joy lies in inspiring them to change their life so they might never again need my invasive angioplasty services.

Throughout my career, I have tried to identify the factors that will help my patients live longer, and importantly, live better. Under the right circumstances, a coronary angioplasty can save a life—and I am ready to intervene if necessary—but I prefer my patients need not undergo this procedure in the first place.

I have always wanted to be a doctor, to use my knowledge to save lives. Even as a child, I can't recall wanting to do anything else. After high school, I gained acceptance into a very competitive accelerated medical program, in which I obtained a bachelor's degree and medical degree in six years instead of the traditional eight, through a program at Rensselaer Polytechnic Institute and Albany Medical College. At the age of 23, I earned my MD.

Initially, I thought emergency medicine might be my calling. The excitement of the acutely sick patient who needs immediate attention thrilled and inspired me. For a brief time during my third year of medical school, I thought about going into family practice, as I observed my preceptor local family doc—who truly got to know his patients within the community—caring for four or even five generations of the same family. Then, hematology struck my interest during a fourth-year medical school rotation at Ben Taub Hospital in Houston, where I saw some of the most interesting blood-related illnesses within an underserved urban population.

Ultimately, I chose a residency in internal medicine, which is the care of the adult patient. I knew that I wanted to treat adults, and I loved the thoughtful, problem-based approach to the patient care of complex illnesses. Also, I had the feeling I might want to specialize in a particular niche of medicine, and training in internal medicine would be prerequisite for any subspecialty.

During my internal medicine residency, the more I was exposed to heart disease, the more my fascination grew. Heart disease was a unique field; so many people develop heart problems, and there is so much research on how to treat it. The interventions that are performed within cardiology—from angioplasties to medicines to lifestyle interventions—make a difference and save lives.

For example, consider a stent placed in a coronary artery in a patient in the throes of a heart attack. Just minutes after the patient's arrival in the emergency room, he is already in a catheterization laboratory, being worked on by a team that opens up his blocked artery and saves his life. I found this type of procedural magic extraordinary.

The evidence upon which heart disease treatment is based fascinated me as well. Of all of the fields of medicine, heart disease has some of the most robust evidence in the research literature surrounding it. In fact, during my residency as I was solidifying my decision to pursue cardiology, I had the opportunity to contribute to this body of knowledge with my own research on heart disease. I studied the importance of the EKG in the prognosis of heart failure patients, and my research was published in the journal *Chest* in August 2002.

My personal background and my approach to the treatment of patients with heart disease are particularly unique. I have extensively studied the role of dietary lifestyle in reducing the risk of heart disease. Many people do not know that a whole-food, plant-based vegan diet can prevent and even reverse the most severe artery blockages, and those who do know this information may be afraid to make such a daunting change to their eating habits. However, a plant-based diet is perhaps the most effective strategy in reversing or reducing one's risk for heart disease, and therefore it must be ranked as an overwhelmingly effective plan. This is the diet that I personally follow and thrive on.

Another component that has shaped my cardiology work is the fact that I am also an endurance athlete, having completed triathlons of all distances, including two Ironman distance triathlons (which consists of a 24-mile swim, a 112-mile bike ride, and a 26.2 mile run), marathons, century cycling rides, and swimming competitions. While I would never expect most of my patients to take on competitive athletics in this extreme manner, I share my enthusiasm for fitness and encourage my patients to follow their own passion for staying fit. (Though one of my former patients—nearly 20 years older than I am—is now a competitive swimmer who has won medals at the United States Senior Games as well as internationally, and can swim circles around me!)

But perhaps the most extraordinary influencing factor that has shaped my journey as a marathon-ing, plant-eating, interventional cardiologist is the fact that I am one of the few cardiologists who has actually been a heart patient herself!

While I do not have coronary artery disease, the most common disease that I treat and the heart issue that I speak of most in this book, I did have a significant abnormal heart rhythm. As a result, I've been a patient on a cardiac catheterization table, when I underwent an invasive ablation procedure that cured me of a nagging cardiac arrhythmia.

It all started in early 2009, when I noticed some seemingly random short bursts of palpitations and lightheadedness. A similar episode occurred later while I was lifting weights, but I hadn't had much sleep the night before and chalked it up to exhaustion. Still, I became concerned enough that I started wearing my heart rate monitor more frequently.

Then during a weight training session, I felt those same symptoms while doing squats. I looked at my heart rate monitor and saw that it read 180 beats per minute. *That can't be right,* I thought. My first instinct was to keep exercising and hope it would stop;

however, doing squats with a racing heart doesn't work so well. I tried carotid sinus massage, pressing on my neck to try to stop the racing heart rhythm. Then I lay down, and by bearing down (also known as a Valsalva maneuver), I was finally able to break the endless loop as my heart rate suddenly slowed down to 73 beats per minute.

Being a cardiologist, I knew that this was likely supraventricular tachycardia—in other words, an abnormal circuit in the heart that can cause the heart to race. My suspicions were proven correct. A few weeks later, while riding my bike, I felt the palpitations again, pulled out a diagnostic heart rhythm monitor that had been prescribed for me, and was able to "record" my racing heart rhythm.

Soon after, I had my ablation procedure at Glendale Memorial Hospital, an organization where I had been on staff for a year and a half. I can still remember how I felt lying there on the table that day. It was a lengthy procedure—about three and a half hours—thanks to my atypical electrical pathway. At times I felt nervous, uncomfortable, vulnerable, and awkward. But this procedure proved to be a very valuable experience for me, and not just because it healed me of my arrhythmia.

While my time as a heart patient was quite brief, it did leave a lasting impression on me and still impacts how I practice medicine to this day. I now know exactly what it feels like to lie on a cath lab table. I know what it is like to be sedated and even feel a bit vulnerable surrounded by machines and technology. Most of all, though, I feel like I can relate to the fear and uncertainty that my patients face as they navigate their heart conditions. I take these experiences with me into the exam room, into the cath lab, and into the hospital ward whenever I treat my patients.

The first section of this book will cover everything you need to know about the heart, and cardiovascular disease, and the various ways it can affect a person's life. You will begin to learn just why the daily choices you make are so important and how wellness is achievable for anyone willing to make a few simple, sensible adjustments. I am honored to be your guide as we set out on this journey together.

CHAPTER 1

The Basics of Cardiology

We are about to take an in-depth look at heart disease as well as all the potential health problems associated with this illness. I'm sure you've already heard a lot about conditions related to heart disease and the very fact that you are reading this book suggests that either you or one of your loved ones may be battling it right now. Still, before we get started, I want to take a moment to share with you some very basic information about how the heart operates.

Also in this chapter we will discuss the role that a cardiologist, like myself, plays in the treatment of heart disease and its various complications. In short, cardiology deals in anything involving the care and wellness of the heart and surrounding blood vessels. We cardiologists are not miracle workers—but we are highly trained technicians who work very hard to educate, inform, and make a difference in our patients' lives.

First, I want to talk about the "heart" of the matter, which is, of course, *your* heart. The heart is arguably the most important organ of the body, and it is crucial in supplying blood to the body, which delivers much-needed oxygen and nutrients to our cells—keeping us alive and well. Before we learn about the various ways and reasons your heart can fail to work properly, it is important to first understand how a healthy heart functions.

Our heart contains four chambers and four valves. The chambers of the heart hold blood, and the valves open and close with each beat of the heart so that blood can pass through. The heart is divided into a left and right side and consists of a right atrium and ventricle, and then a left atrium and ventricle. The atria of the heart act as collecting chambers, while the ventricles of the heart are the muscular chambers that pump blood throughout the body. There are four valves, the tricuspid, pulmonic, mitral, and aortic, which open and close to allow blood to pass.

Blood returns to the heart through blood vessels called veins. The two largest veins of the body, the superior and inferior vena cava, deliver blood to the right atrium of the heart. The tricuspid valve, which separates the right atrium and right ventricle, opens and blood empties from the atrium into the ventricle. Then, the right ventricle squeezes, pushing blood through the pulmonic valve, and into the main pulmonary artery, and then into the smaller pulmonary arteries, which are the arteries of the lungs.

Blood travels to the small vessels of the lungs, called capillaries, and then to the alveoli of the lungs, where blood becomes oxygenated. Then, this oxygen-rich blood returns to the heart through four pulmonary veins to the left atrium. The mitral valve opens, and blood passes to the left ventricle. From here, the left ventricle squeezes blood across the aortic valve, into the aorta, and from there it flows to the organs and tissues of the body.

The process I have described above illustrates the functioning of a normal, healthy heart. However, there are many disease processes that can cause the heart's function to go awry. This can range from abnormalities occurring in the structure of the walls or valves of the heart, the electrical system of the heart, or in the supply of blood to the heart muscle itself.

What Is Coronary Artery Disease?

The heart is made up of muscle. Each time the heart beats, several millions of muscle fibers contract, allowing blood to move through the heart. Since the heart itself is a muscle, the heart requires its own source of blood in order to function. Coronary arteries are the vessels that supply the heart muscle with blood. When the lining of those vessels becomes filled with a waxy substance called plaque, the result is known as coronary artery disease.

You may be wondering what could lead to an artery getting clogged up. It certainly isn't a natural part of aging. Risk factors for coronary artery disease include high blood pressure, elevated cholesterol, diabetes, poor diet, family history, age, a sedentary lifestyle, and cigarette smoke. We will discuss these issues in more detail later in the book. While some risk factors, such as family history, cannot be changed, most risk factors can be modified, managed, or even alleviated.

Angina, which is heart-related chest pain or shortness of breath, occurs when an insufficient amount of blood reaches the heart muscle. In other words, the heart muscle tissue is temporarily starved of oxygen, leading to the above symptoms.

This often occurs with exertion or exercise, because when the body is working harder physically, the heart must work harder and faster to supply oxygenated blood to the body. In most cases, angina is related to a significant narrowing of a coronary artery due to coronary artery disease, through there are other less common causes of angina such as coronary artery spasm or inherited abnormalities of the coronary arteries.

What Is a Heart Attack?

A heart attack is a sudden event in which the flow of blood to a portion of the heart is abruptly cut off, and, as a result, heart muscle tissue dies. The most common cause of a heart attack is a piece of plaque suddenly rupturing from the wall of a coronary artery and immediately blocking an artery completely, which stops the flow of blood to portions of the heart distal to that point.

The most common symptoms of a heart attack are chest pain, shortness of breath, sweating, left arm or jaw pain, nausea, and vomiting. However, less common symptoms can occur, more frequently in women, such as back pain, fatigue, or lightheadedness.

You must be aware that a heart attack is a medical emergency. The longer the heart muscle is starved of oxygen, the more heart muscle dies, and the more likely that one may have significant permanent damage to the heart. Further, a heart attack can lead to a cardiac arrest, an abnormal heart rhythm that causes the heart to completely stop pumping, and can lead to death within minutes if CPR is not started immediately.

What Is a Stroke?

A stroke, similar to a heart attack, occurs when blood flow to a portion of the brain is suddenly cut off. Typically, this occurs in the same manner as a heart attack, in that a piece of plaque from the artery breaks off, usually from one of the carotid arteries supplying the brain, and completely occludes an artery of the brain distally, cutting off blood flow to that portion of the brain. Another common cause of a stroke is a clot traveling from the heart to the brain, often due to an arrhythmia called atrial

What Should You Do If You Think You Are Having a Heart Attack or Stroke?

If you suspect you are having a heart attack or a stroke, the smartest course of action is to call 911 immediately. Do not ask someone to drive you to the hospital, or worse yet drive yourself; that can delay care and can be downright dangerous. By calling 911, you are activating an emergency response system, starting with the trained medical professionals who can immediately start assessing and treating you. The emergency medical professionals can also make sure to take you to an appropriate hospital that has the facilities to treat your condition.

13

fibrillation, or due to another structural abnormality of the heart. Symptoms can include sudden onset weakness or numbness of one side of the face or body, slurred speech, change in vision, difficulty with balance or walking, or confusion.

How Do Doctors Treat Coronary Artery Disease?

Doctors are able to treat coronary artery disease with medications. Aspirin therapy can reduce the risk of a heart attack or stroke in appropriately selected patients. Statin medications can lower cholesterol levels, help stabilize plaque, and reduce the risk of a heart attack or stroke. Other medications, such as beta blockers, calcium channel blockers, or nitrates, can help improve blood flow through tightly blocked arteries.

There are also more invasive ways of treating coronary artery disease, either with angioplasty or with bypass surgery. In the case of certain types of heart attacks, these procedures can save a life. Otherwise, and in most cases, they do not prolong life or reduce the risk of a heart attack, and their role is primarily to improve blood flow and reduce angina symptoms.

Angioplasty is a procedure in which coronary artery blockages can be opened up from outside of the body. A sheath, or a large tube, is placed in either the common femoral artery in the groin area, or in the radial artery at the wrist. A catheter is fed up through the artery, into the aorta, and inserted into the opening of one of the major coronary arteries. Dye is then injected through the catheter into the coronary arteries, and X-ray pictures can be taken to view the outline of the arteries. If a significant blockage is identified, then a wire is passed through the blockage, a balloon is advanced along the wire, and then inflates. This balloon expands the artery and shifts plaque out of the way. Next, a stent, which is a tiny metal scaffolding, is placed at this location to hold the artery open.

Coronary artery bypass surgery is far more invasive than angioplasty. A cardiothoracic surgeon cuts the chest open and then bypasses blockages. He or she does not clean out the arteries, but rather uses veins and arteries from other parts of the body to reroute blood around these severe blockages. Bypass surgery usually entails a stay in the hospital of five days on average, and recovery time is several weeks, if not months.

A cardiologist's goal is to stop or reverse the progression of coronary artery disease. In order to accomplish this, we must get to the root of the problem—treat elevated blood pressure, lower elevated cholesterol levels, control diabetes, quit smoking, make healthy food choices, exercise, lose excess weight, and manage stress. Later on, we will talk about how you can make changes that can ultimately halt or even reverse heart disease.

Now that you've learned a bit about the heart muscle and the role that your cardiologist can play in maintaining your health, we are ready to delve deeply into the various ways that heart disease can manifest, along with the known precursors of coronary artery disease. In the next chapter, we will take an in-depth look at heart disease, diabetes, hypertension, and cholesterol, as well as what you can do to make the most of your doctor's visits. We will also cover the types of surgery that may be necessary if your condition progresses past a certain point.

Later in the book, I will lay out my proven plan that explains how your diet and lifestyle can best help you manage and even reverse some of the symptoms of coronary artery disease. I will show you the way to make the best health choices and improve your quality of life. I want you to know that there is hope and that you have an opportunity ahead of you to take control of your health, starting right now.

CHAPTER 2

The Risk Factors for Heart Disease

Many people live in fear that they will develop heart disease. And for good reason: Unhealthy lifestyles abound, and heart disease is often the cumulative result of years of bad choices and bad habits. Coronary artery disease, heart attacks, and strokes don't just "happen." Damaging plaque builds up slowly over the course of many years. Blood pressure levels slowly elevate, and cholesterol rises as we make yet another bad dietary choice.

Of course, there is a genetic component to heart disease, and we can't control and prevent everything. But there's plenty we *can* do to improve the odds—"we" meaning doctors and patients alike—and it's never too late to start. Doctors have the experience and technology to monitor the precursors of coronary artery disease in their patients. We can help our patients by prescribing the best medicines for their conditions. And patients, each day, have the choice to acknowledge their risk for coronary artery disease and take steps to prevent it.

In this chapter, I will discuss the known risk factors for heart disease. Remember, I am still "setting the stage" for the actionable advice that will come later in this book. I believe knowledge is power, and being educated on the important issues surrounding heart disease will only strengthen your resolve to get healthy now.

Know What You CAN'T Change—and Change What You CAN

There are several risk factors for heart disease. Some of these risk factors can be modified to lower a person's chances of developing heart disease, and, unfortunately, others cannot. For example, age and gender are two risk factors for heart disease that cannot be controlled. The older you are, the more time you have had to accumulate damage to your body and your arteries. Also, men have a higher risk of heart disease, and they tend to develop it at a younger age than women. (However, after women go through menopause, their risk for heart disease increases and narrows this gender gap.)

Having a family history of heart disease is another risk factor that cannot be modified. If your parents or siblings have coronary artery disease, particularly at a young age, your own risk is increased. This may be related to genetic abnormalities, but it is important to keep in mind that members of the same family may have similar bad lifestyle habits that also increase risk. That said, even if you have many family members who have had heart problems at a young age does *not* mean you are destined to meet the same fate. By concentrating on the changes you can make, you can live free of heart problems for decades.

And yes, there are some critical risk factors that you do have the power to modify. These include smoking, living a sedentary lifestyle, and being overweight or obese. *You can* quit smoking, *you can* choose to exercise, and *you can* eat a healthy diet so you are able to lose weight. That's a lot of power in your hands, and it is my fervent hope that you will use it to better your present and lengthen your future. (We will talk more about these crucial lifestyle changes later in the book.)

Our lives are *made* by the choices we make each day, and each of us live by our thoughts and actions. We choose what we focus on moment to moment. It is important for you to realize that you can prevent further damage to your heart *right now*, by choosing to modify your behavior. Sure, you can also choose to wring your hands and resign yourself to having a heart attack at 55, like your father did. Or you can decide to make better choices today, to fix your diet, quit smoking, and get active. There is no down side (at all!) to fixing bad nutritional and lifestyle habits. By making these healthy changes, you will look and feel better, have more energy, and, most importantly, *you* will be the captain of your life. Not coronary artery disease.

All that said, there are several health conditions, which, if managed properly, can greatly reduce your risk of developing heart disease, particularly hypertension (high blood pressure), high cholesterol, and diabetes. Again, in the interest of educating yourself and getting the lay of the land, let's discuss each one.

THE VEGAN HEART DOCTOR'S GUIDE

Understanding Blood Pressure and Hypertension

Your blood pressure describes the measurement of the force applied against the walls of the arteries as your heart pumps blood throughout the body. The systolic blood pressure, or top number of a blood pressure reading, is the highest amount of pressure that the arteries experience, which occurs right after the left ventricle chamber of the heart squeezes blood. The diastolic blood pressure is the lower number of a blood pressure reading, and is the measure of pressure within the arteries when the heart is relaxed and is not squeezing blood.

A normal blood pressure result is considered to be 120/80 or less. Hypertension, or high blood pressure, is classified as a blood pressure reading of 130/80 or higher, based on recent guidelines released in 2017. Hypertension can also exist when one of these numbers, either the systolic or the diastolic, is high and the other is normal.

The Causes of High Blood Pressure

There are many factors that can affect a person's blood pressure: the amount of water and salt in the body; the condition of the nervous system, kidneys, and blood vessels; hormone levels; and finally, stress.

As people get older, their systolic blood pressure levels tend to rise. Other factors that can increase the risk of hypertension include being African-American, obesity, high levels of stress or anxiety, drinking too much alcohol (more than one drink a day for women and two drinks a day for men), untreated sleep apnea, a diet high in sodium, family history of high blood pressure, diabetes, and smoking.

Factors That Put You at Risk for Hypertension

- Obesity
- Stress and anxiety
- Too much alcohol
- Untreated sleep apnea
- A high-sodium diet
- Family history of hypertension
- Diabetes
- Smoking
- Being African-American

The Scope of the Problem

One in every three American adults has hypertension. And, unfortunately, only half of those have their blood pressure under control.[1] As a result, more than 360,000 deaths in the United States in 2013 included high blood pressure as a primary or contributing cause. That is 1,000 deaths each day.[2]

African-Americans have the highest risk of hypertension, with 43 percent of African-American men and 45.7 percent of African-American women having hypertension. On the other hand, Mexican-Americans have a lower incidence of hypertension, with 27.8 percent and 28.9 percent of men and women, respectively, having hypertension.[3]

In 2009, there were 55 million visits to healthcare providers in the United States for hypertension. Sadly, about one in five adults with hypertension are not aware that they have high blood pressure, leading to many of the complications associated with uncontrolled hypertension.[4]

How Hypertension Is Diagnosed

Blood pressure is measured using an inflatable arm cuff with a gauge. This measurement should be taken with the patient seated calmly, in a chair, back resting on the back of the chair, ankles and legs uncrossed with feet flat on the ground, and the arm supported at heart level. Keeping in mind that the blood pressure fluctuates from minute to minute, a single elevated blood pressure reading should not lead to an instant diagnosis of hypertension, but rather should be confirmed with repeated blood pressure measurements on different days.

The Impact of Untreated Hypertension

Hypertension is often referred to as the "silent killer." Most people with uncontrolled hypertension do not even have symptoms. Over time, their bodies become accustomed to the elevated pressures within the arteries. And yet, at the same time, those elevated pressures are damaging the arteries, the heart, and the organs of the body.

Uncontrolled high blood pressure leads to an enlargement of the heart. As the heart muscle has to generate extra force to pump blood through higher pressure arteries, it thickens, just as when we lift heavy weights our skeletal muscles get bigger. Hypertension also causes stiffness of the heart and makes it difficult for the heart muscle to relax. It also leads to increasing the burden of plaque in the arteries and the consequences of coronary disease. Also, all of these effects can increase the risk of congestive heart failure, a condition in which the heart is overwhelmed by the volume of fluid that it has to pump.

Ultimately, uncontrolled hypertension has dire consequences, including increased risk of heart attack and stroke, congestive heart failure, the heart rhythm abnormality called atrial fibrillation, kidney disease, erectile dysfunction, peripheral artery disease, vision problems, and memory loss.

How to Lower Blood Pressure Naturally

Blood pressure is affected by a person's lifestyle. A diet that is high in sodium will raise the blood pressure. Choosing to eat more fruits and vegetables and less animal products will lower the blood pressure. A plant-based diet is a very potent way to lower blood pressure; in fact, in the 1940s, before blood pressure medications were available, Dr. Walter Kempner was the first doctor to successfully lower blood pressure, which he accomplished with a very strict fruit and rice diet. Weight loss and regular exercise are also excellent ways to control hypertension. If a patient's blood pressure is only mildly elevated, I will try a lifestyle approach before I suggest adding medications. Many people can control their blood pressure well by improving the diet, exercising regularly, and losing a few pounds.

Controlling Your Blood Pressure

Blood pressure control with medications is much a process of trial and error. Often it takes a few attempts to find medications that don't have side effects and that are well tolerated. Your doctor can help you find the best blood pressure medication for you, so be up front and report whether you are experiencing unpleasant side effects.

My own approach to blood pressure control often involves several office visits. We will discuss diet, exercise, weight loss, stress management. Slowly, I will add or increase the dose of blood pressure medications at each visit. I work slowly, because my greatest fear, especially in an elderly patient, is to overmedicate someone and cause her to be lightheaded and at risk of falling. After several visits, ultimately, we will work together and get blood pressure under control. That said, blood pressure medications are never permanent. If, over time, a patient eats better, exercises more, and loses weight, the blood pressure naturally comes down, and together we can decrease and even eliminate medications.

Cholesterol: The Good (HDL), the Bad (LDL), and the Fatty (Triglycerides)

Cholesterol is produced by our liver and is necessary for our body to function appropriately. It builds and maintains the outer layer of the cells of the body, helps produce our hormones, metabolizes vitamins, and insulates our nerve fibers.

We get cholesterol from two sources: what our body produces and what we eat. Our bodies make more than enough cholesterol for our bodies to function. Since animals, like us, synthesize cholesterol, when we eat animal products, we are consuming cholesterol. Vegan diets, therefore, are naturally cholesterol-free. However, just because a food is vegan does not necessarily mean it is a healthy choice for the heart or for cholesterol. Processed foods, whether vegan or not, that may be higher in saturated and trans-fats, can raise your cholesterol levels.

When we have our "cholesterol checked," we are not having our actual cholesterol particles measured. Instead, doctors measure your lipoproteins, which are the lipid particles that function to transport cholesterol. They are:

- **LDL: low-density lipoprotein**—This is known as the "bad" cholesterol. LDL transports cholesterol from the liver to cells. As a result, patients with high levels of LDL cholesterol have a higher risk of heart disease, and lower LDL is associated with a lower risk of heart disease.

- **HDL: high-density lipoprotein**—This is known as the "good" cholesterol. HDL performs the opposite function of LDL. It carries cholesterol from the cells of the body back to the liver. People with higher levels of HDL tend to have a lower risk of coronary disease. On the other hand, those people with lower levels of HDL are at higher risk of heart disease. HDL cholesterol levels should ideally be higher than 40 in men and higher than 50 in women.

- **Triglycerides**—Most fat found in our food, as well as in the body, exists in the form of triglycerides. In addition to triglycerides coming from fats in our food, they are also made from other energy sources, such as excess carbohydrates. Calories ingested and not used immediately by our tissues are converted to triglycerides and transported to our fat cells to be stored. Being overweight and physically inactive can lead to high triglyceride levels—as can cigarette smoking and excess alcohol consumption.

Also, certain diseases, medications, or genetic disorders can be the cause of elevated triglyceride levels. Elevated triglyceride levels are linked to coronary artery disease and can even cause pancreatitis, which is inflammation of the pancreas.

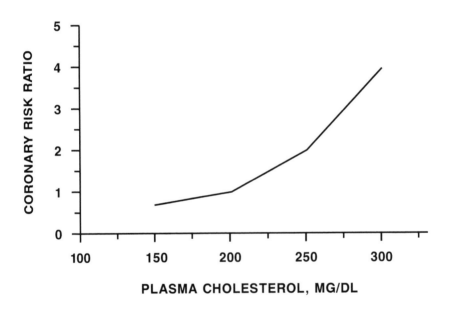

Table 1: Higher total cholesterol levels are linked to increased risk of coronary disease[5]

According to the American Heart Association, what your cholesterol levels should be:[6]

LDL Cholesterol Levels	
Less than 100 mg/dL	Optimal
100 to 129 mg/dL	Near Optimal/Above Optimal
130 to 159 mg/dL	Borderline High
160 to 189 mg/dL	High
190 mg/dL and above	Very High

Triglyceride levels:

- Normal: less than 150 mg/dL
- Borderline High: 150 to 199 mg/dL
- High: 200 to 499 mg/dL
- Very High: 500 mg/dL

Treating Abnormal Cholesterol

The most recent guidelines on treatment of cholesterol to lower the risk of heart disease were released in late 2013, and with plenty of controversy. Much like the treatment of high blood pressure, the first line of treatment for abnormal cholesterol levels is to implement lifestyle change. However, certain patients, particularly those at higher risk of heart disease and those already diagnosed with heart disease, are often treated with cholesterol lowering medication. These medications are known as statins.[7]

Statins are the preferred medication for elevated cholesterol. Statins are not only very effective at lowering cholesterol, but they also have beneficial effects on the artery linings, stabilize plaque, and can lead to reversal of coronary artery disease.[8] Statins are most potent in reducing the risk of heart attack or stroke in people who have already had these events, but can also reduce cardiovascular risk in those who have never had an event.[9, 10] The older statins, like pravastatin and lovastatin are less potent, while newer statins such as atorvastatin (Lipitor), rosuvastatin (Crestor), and pitavastatin (Livalo) are stronger.

If you have already had a heart attack or stroke, a coronary stent, or carry a diagnosis of coronary artery disease or peripheral artery disease, there is strong evidence that a statin will reduce your risk of recurrent events, regardless of how low your cholesterol numbers are. If you have high cholesterol and have not had one of these events, but have other risk factors like diabetes, hypertension, or severely elevated cholesterol, you may also benefit from a statin. An informed discussion with your doctor is important in deciding whether a statin medication is appropriate.

Understanding Diabetes

Diabetes is a condition in which the body does not metabolize glucose correctly, and it is a known strong risk factor for coronary artery disease. When you eat, your body turns food into sugar, also known as glucose. Glucose is broken down by insulin so that it can be used for energy. If there is not enough insulin, or the tissues are not sensitive to insulin, then blood sugar levels will rise, and damage to the body can occur.

There are two types of diabetes: type 1 and type 2. Type 1 diabetes is the less common form of diabetes. It tends to occur in younger patients and is thought to be due to a process that destroys the pancreas, the organ responsible for making insulin. Type 2 diabetes, on the other hand, is far more common, typically occurs in older patients, and is a condition in which the body is less sensitive to insulin, leading to increases in blood glucose levels.

It is not always the case that young people have type 1 diabetes and older people have type 2 diabetes. Older patients can develop type 1 diabetes, but this occurs less often. On the other hand, younger, particularly obese people, can develop type 2 diabetes.

The only way to treat type 1 diabetes is with insulin therapy. On the other hand, glucose levels can be controlled in type 2 diabetes with pills, insulin, or a combination of pills and insulin. That said, lifestyle goes a long way to help control blood sugars, just as it does with blood pressure and cholesterol levels.

By far, the most common cause of diabetes is the type 2 variety—insulin resistance. Though it is growing more prevalent, type 2 diabetes is very much preventable. Maintaining a healthy body weight, exercising, and eating a healthy diet greatly reduces the risk of developing this type of diabetes.

Consequences of Uncontrolled Diabetes

Controlling blood glucose levels is absolutely critical in managing diabetes. Diabetes greatly increases your risk of heart attack and stroke, but diabetes affects many other organ systems as well. It is the most common cause of blindness, kidney failure, and amputations. Diabetes can also cause neuropathy, which is dysfunction and damage to the nerves in the body. Peripheral neuropathy can lead to nerve damage to the feet and hands, resulting in lack of sensation and, in some people, chronic pain.

Autonomic neuropathy affects the nerves that control our internal organs; this can cause gastroparesis (which refers to decreased motility of the gut), sexual problems, dizziness and fainting, and difficulty in sensing when your bladder is full.

Heart disease is a particular concern for diabetics, as diabetes increases the risk of heart attack and stroke. In fact, two out of three diabetics will die of heart attack or stroke. When diabetes is combined with other risk factors, like smoking, uncontrolled hypertension, and hyperlipidemia, the risk of heart disease skyrockets.

I've talked about the risk factors for heart disease and the consequences if they are not controlled, but there is hope. By working with your doctor to control your risk factors, taking the right medications if needed, eating well and exercising, you can thrive. If you have not yet had a heart problem, you can greatly reduce your risk just by paying attention to your lifestyle choices. Even if you have already suffered a heart attack or stroke, by taking control of your health, you can live healthier and longer than you may have imagined.

As your wellness journey continues, you will no doubt have plenty of appointments with various specialists as well as your general practitioner. Up next, we will be talking about how you can make the most of your visits with your medical team. By being a great patient, you can receive the utmost level of care from each doctor you visit.

CHAPTER 3

How to Be a Good Patient

Let me begin this chapter by stating that there is no substitute for assuming responsibility for your well-being. Taking good care of yourself is critical, and only you can decide to be proactive about your health. However: In addition to making wise day-to-day decisions, it is important that you commit to visiting the appropriate doctors for your particular health needs.

That said, if you have a history of heart issues, it is essential that you enlist the watchful eye of your cardiologist from time to time. Cardiologists are highly trained specialists who understand the ins and outs of heart disease and they can guide you on your journey toward wellness. I've put together some of my thoughts, gleaned from my perspective as a physician, on how to get the most from your specialist's guidance.

Some of this guidance may seem like common sense, and some of it may be less obvious, but these are all things that I see on a day-to-day basis. In my years of practice, I have dealt both with disorganized, apathetic patients as well as those who were totally on top of their game. It is my experience that the patients who come to their appointments prepared and eager to heal get the most benefit from their physician's guidance.

The lesson is clear: When you are prepared, engaged, and well-informed, you can get so much more out of your interactions with your doctor.

Getting Prepared for a Visit

Know your history before you set off for the doctor's office. This is particularly important if this is your first visit to a new cardiologist. The office can get records, but often there is a delay, or pertinent records are missing. However, you can establish a written record of not only *your* medical history, but also your family history as well as medications you have taken in the past up until now.

Before you leave for your visit, jot down any notes you can remember in a notebook or on your smartphone. Carry this information with you each time you visit your cardiologist and any other doctors you meet with. This notebook will become your "health journal," and it will help keep you organized. Writing it all down prior to your visit is so important because you may forget important questions or info when you're "on the spot." Trust me, this happens to everyone—myself included—so it's better to err on the side of caution and come with a list in hand. Furthermore, doctors unfortunately have a limited amount of time to meet with their patients, so keeping a notebook handy helps you relay all the pertinent information in an efficient manner.

Know Your Medications

You may have memorized all the medications you take daily just out of habit. However, don't rely on your memory to serve you accurately during a visit with your cardiologist. Keep a list of medications and doses with you so you will be sure to give your doctor the correct information. It is also helpful to grab all of your pill bottles, even if there are a lot of them, and bring them to the doctor's office. Another strategy is to use your

Your Heart History Checklist

It is important to know your heart history so you can convey it to your cardiologist and your entire medical team. Here is a checklist of information your doctors will need to be aware of.

• Have you seen a cardiologist in the past few years? What is his or her name?

• Have you been hospitalized recently? If so, where and for what?

• Have you had a heart attack? How long ago? At what hospital were you cared for?

• Have you had an angioplasty? Do you have any coronary stents in place? If so, do you have the wallet cards that should have been given to you at the time of your procedure?

• Have you had heart surgery? Where was it performed, and what type of surgery was performed?

• Do you have a pacemaker or defibrillator? If so, do you have the wallet card from the manufacturer with information about the device? (Be sure to keep this card in your wallet or purse.)

smartphone to take a picture of the front of all of your pill bottles and show this to your doctor.

It is incorrect to assume that what is "in the chart" is sufficient, or to state that you are "on the same meds as before." Mistakes happen often, and you simply can't count on accurate records to be taken at every single juncture of your wellness journey. Only you know what medication bottles you have at home and what pills you take every day. All too often, patients will be prescribed medications by other providers that are inappropriate, or a patient may forget to pick up a medicine from the pharmacy, and mistakes like these lead to an inaccurate list of medications in the chart.

Take charge of your health by coming prepared with a list of what you are currently taking and what you have taken in the past. Furthermore, make a note of any medications to which you are allergic or have reacted badly in the past. This is important information for your doctor, as she may need to make additional adjustments to your medications.

Make sure that you have completed any testing that may have been ordered by the doctor prior to your appointment. If blood work was requested, have it done a few days before the appointment so that the results will be ready in time.

Bring with you any information that may have been requested prior to the office visit. Often, I will ask a patient to check his blood pressure at home and keep a list of the blood pressure readings. Or, I may ask a patient to bring in her home blood pressure cuff so we can compare the reading of her home machine to what we obtain with our blood pressure cuff in the office to make sure that her machine works properly.

Know the issues you want to discuss with your cardiologist today. Make sure that your main concern for that visit is addressed with the medical assistant who brings you to the exam room. My medical assistant will let me know, before I come in the room, what your main concern is, which may prompt me to review records of yours that may be pertinent.

If your main concern is your chest pain, for example, bring that up first when the doctor enters the room. While as a cardiologist I care about you as a whole, and not just your heart, a lengthy description of your recent frustrations with knee pain is going to take away from the time that I can spend in helping your heart condition.

And it's always challenging at the end of a visit, when I ask if there is anything else I can do—and after spending the entire visit discussing a plan to improve leg swelling—the patient asks, "What about my chest pain?" Be sure to bring up all health concerns *before* the meeting comes to an end.

During the Visit

It is so important that you show up on time to your doctor's appointment. If it is a first visit, you may be asked to come in early to fill out paperwork. Being prompt will help ensure that you are calm and relaxed for your visit; further, your doctor will be less rushed and can take the appropriate amount of time to speak with and properly treat you.

While it may seem like common sense, try to eliminate any distractions during your visit. Turn off your cell phone. Nothing interrupts the flow of an important conversation more than a repeatedly ringing or chiming mobile device. Also, try not to bring anyone who might be a distraction, such as a young child whose behavior you may not be able to predict.

If you are concerned about remembering what you are told, or are not sure that you can convey what you need to say to your doctor, have a family member or friend with you. Don't forget that you can also take notes in your notebook or on your smartphone to ensure that you remember all that you need to.

Try to be fully engaged when meeting with your cardiologist. A patient who seems interested will truly get the most out of his visit to the doctor. Appropriate questions not only clarify your own uncertainties, but engaging your physician in a conversation will provide more information and discussion of your condition.

Listen closely, take notes if you feel you need to, and make sure you understand what your doctor tells you. Even if you are stressed, confused, or upset due to receiving bad news, it is very important to stay focused during your appointment. If you do not understand something that has been said, don't be afraid to ask questions to clarify. I know that many patients feel afraid to bombard their doctors with lots of questions, but don't be. This "back and forth" dynamic is crucial to a doctor/patient relationship. Your doctor should be happy to comply.

And just a word on bringing in your own health-related research: Sometimes patients share with me information they have discovered on their own; perhaps advice from a family member or a neighbor, or something they've read on the internet. Some of this may be good advice, but much of it may not be. Feel free to discuss this information with your doctor so that you don't walk away from your appointment with any misconceptions about your health.

If your doctor wants you to undergo any testing, make sure you understand all the pertinent information regarding those tests. It is important to understand why the tests are requested, where the testing will be done, and finally, any instructions for how to prepare for the test (such as whether or not you should be eating anything or taking your medications on the morning of the test).

If your doctor prescribes a new medication, make sure you understand the instructions. If your doctor hand-writes prescriptions, be sure that you walk out of the office with a prescription in your hand. If your doctor sends prescriptions electronically to the pharmacy, as many of us do, check that he or she knows what pharmacy to send your prescription to and what quantity of medications to request. Be ready to tell your doctor whether you would like a 30-day or 90-day supply of your prescription.

After the Visit

Sometimes, after a visit, questions can arise. You may not completely understand the instructions you were given. A new medication may be causing you to feel unwell. Or, you may be having difficulty in scheduling a test that was ordered by your doctor.

Any of these would be appropriate reasons to call your doctor's office. It is frustrating to see a patient back in a couple months to assess his progress only to find out that he didn't have a needed test done or stopped a medication just two days after it was prescribed.

Any new symptom that comes up between appointments can be concerning as well. For example, if you start having chest pain every time you exercise, this is something that should not wait. If you have any hesitation at all about your symptoms, call your doctor right away! It may be a big nothing, but it is better to know for certain and remain safe.

Why Following Up and Ongoing Care Are Important

If you have heart disease, you should be seeing your cardiologist regularly. Even if you are feeling fine, it is good to touch base, just to make sure that everything is in check. There are some situations in which regular cardiologist visits are absolutely vital. For example, if you've had a coronary stent placed, a bypass surgery, or have had a heart attack, you absolutely should be following up with your doctor regularly. After any one of these events, you are at an increased risk of future problems. Regular visits with your cardiologist can help prevent additional trauma and can monitor your current state of health.

At a return visit, your cardiologist will follow up on your condition. If I were your physician, I would review medications, labs (including cholesterol levels), and assess your progress. We would also talk about your lifestyle habits and whether you are having any symptoms. We would discuss which changes—whether they be to medications or lifestyle—could help you to further reduce your risk of future heart problems and live a better and healthier life.

All too often, a patient with heart disease does not get the follow-up with a cardiologist that he or she needs. It is of utmost importance that you return for these subsequent visits, as requested by your cardiologist. No doctor can force patients to follow up after they undergo a surgical procedure or suffer a heart attack. But it is absolutely vital that *you* understand that failure to attend follow-up appointments could have damaging consequences.

The unfortunate truth is that many people who don't follow up with their medical team will suffer progression of their heart disease, heart attacks, strokes, or even premature death unnecessarily.

I can't stress enough the importance of being proactive in your role as a heart disease patient. Doctors, including your cardiologist, are here to help you on your health journey, but *you* are ultimately responsible for your own care. Don't think that by seeing a doctor once a year, you've "done your part." We can't fix your heart disease if you don't follow our advice and actively comply by improving your lifestyle per our instructions.

In most cases your health is the culmination of a lifetime of choices you have made. For many years you have chosen to eat certain foods, exercise (or not), smoke cigarettes (or not), get a certain amount of sleep, and so forth—and now it is time to change the way you've been living. It won't be easy but it absolutely will be worth the effort.

So here's the bottom line: Work with your doctor to keep a two-way channel of communication going. Keep in touch, keep good records, and keep your chin up on your journey to better health. And carefully read the upcoming chapters where we will really dive into the importance of your lifestyle, what you eat, and how much you move as you strive to get—and stay—healthier and happier.

CHAPTER 4

Making a Major Lifestyle Change: How You Can Reclaim Your Life and Health

Armed with the knowledge that true wellness is inextricably linked to our diet and lifestyle, it's easy for us to see that we need to make changes in order to regain our health and really thrive. However, making those changes can seem downright overwhelming at first.

Most cardiology patients know what they need to change in order to reclaim their health and energy. They know that they should be eating better and exercising more that they should stop smoking, and in many cases, also lose some weight. Even if they don't know exactly what they need to do, they understand that they need to make *some kind* of a big change in their lives.

But, how does one go from recognizing a need for dramatic change to taking action?

This is a question most people have struggled with at some point in life. Whether we need to lose weight, get organized, clean a perpetually messy house, change careers, end a bad relationship, or make some other big change, most of us know from experience that old habits die hard. Yet we *can* break destructive patterns—and the patterns that create and perpetuate heart disease are no exception. One of my patients, Harold, is living proof of this.

Harold came to my office for a consultation about five years ago. He was 55 years old, overweight, and on medications for his high blood pressure. He was concerned because every time he would exert himself physically, he would get pressure in his chest. I put him through a stress test, which demonstrated severe abnormalities, and then a coronary angiogram revealed a severe 95 percent narrowing of his left circumflex coronary artery.

I wasted no time in placing a coronary stent into his artery. Then, as I do with all patients, I discussed with Harold measures to improve his health, including starting a healthy plant-based diet and a regular exercise routine. Harold went home and conducted some research on his own, during which time he read Dr. Caldwell Esselstyn's book *Prevent and Reverse Heart Disease* and watched the documentary film *Forks Over Knives*. Following these revelations, he adopted a plant-based diet and began cycling regularly for exercise.

The results were impressive (but not surprising). Harold lost 40 pounds, which he has maintained today, and no longer needs any blood pressure medication. Over these four years, he has remained on a plant-based diet and stuck to a regular exercise routine. Given his starting point of being overweight, medicated, and experiencing a coronary blockage, Harold has done remarkably well. He feels better than he has in many years, and has experienced no further heart issues.

Surprisingly, or perhaps not so surprisingly, it's five years later and Harold still maintains a healthy plant-based diet, rides his bicycle outdoors, and attends a spin class regularly. I asked him what keeps him motivated to stick to these good habits. He said, "I'm a guinea pig for my children. Since they have inherited my genetics, we'll see if what I'm doing works, and if it works for me, it will work for them."

Of all of my patients, Harold is certainly one of the most motivated. Through making substantial, sustainable lifestyle changes, he has been able to heal. I applaud him for taking charge of his health in such a proactive way. However, most people aren't quite that self-motivated. Most of us need a little guidance before we upend our diets and our daily routines. So, what makes us decide to change our ways, to move away from convenient habits that harm our health, and instead adopt health-promoting lifestyle choices?

Doug Lisle, PhD, and Alan Goldhamer, DC, wrote a book called *The Pleasure Trap*, which addresses how we as a society have evolved to the conveniences provided in our high-tech society and how we can make better choices. The book explains that we are motivated by our biological purpose in life, which is survival and, ultimately, reproduction. There are three incentives to fulfill this purpose: the pursuit of pleasure, the avoidance of pain, and the conservation of energy. This is referred to as "The Motivation Triad."

However, this triad can motivate people to make choices that don't necessarily help to preserve our health, a tendency known as "the pleasure trap." The pleasure trap is especially pervasive in modern times, when unhealthy foods abound and when we have the option of spending lazy days on the couch streaming TV shows. Take for example the choice to eat a fast food hamburger. No doubt about it: This is a pleasurable food to eat (for many people, anyway), it very quickly alleviates the pain of hunger (we can start soothing our growling tummy even as we drive), and it conserves our energy because all we need to do is pull up to the drive-thru window.

In the long run, though, eating fast food is a choice that is *not* going to help us to live well or survive. Similarly, drugs of addiction do the same thing; they give us pleasure and keep us from feeling pain in exchange for very little effort on our part.

Our bodies evolved to survive during times when food was scarce. In fact, in much of the world, people living in developing countries still die of starvation today. However, this is definitely no longer our reality in America. We live in a society of abundance, and the diseases that cause death in the Western world are not those of deficiency, but instead are diseases of abundance.

Heart disease, stroke, diabetes, and cancer—the major killers in our society—arise from an overabundance of processed foods that are unnaturally dense in calories. Still, however, our genetic code—which is wired to allow us to survive a famine—leads us to prefer calorie-dense processed and animal foods, *and* to conserve our energy at the same time. Ironically, living in an era when we can have rich, calorie-laden food any time we wish is a dangerous proposition. No, we won't be eaten by a sabre-toothed tiger—but we might be taken down by obesity and an overstressed heart.

Speaking of Obesity...How Does Weight Loss Fit in to Your Return to Health?

Later in this chapter we are going to talk about how you can actually implement the changes necessary to fight coronary artery disease and regain your health and energy. But first, I want to touch on obesity. Many of you reading this book may be overweight. Obesity is certainly a big problem afflicting many people today. Not only does it contribute to heart disease, but it is also a factor in several other dangerous or debilitating conditions like diabetes, chronic joint pain, and back pain—not to mention the psychological turmoil and stigma that comes with carrying too much weight.

Yes, obesity is a dangerous, expensive, and sometimes heartbreaking (literally and figuratively) condition that requires attention and action. However, I want to be clear that this is *not* a book about weight loss. Getting thin is not your primary goal in taking back your health; instead the goal is to heal your heart and put you safely out of the danger zone for heart disease.

Nonetheless, as you start incorporating the changes described in this book and embrace a new lifestyle geared toward improving your health and vitality, you most likely *will* lose weight. But in this context, your weight loss will occur as an organic and happy side effect. Luckily for everyone, making your heart happy and making your body fit and capable go hand in hand.

Let's try to grasp the scope of today's obesity epidemic. About two-thirds of people in our country are overweight, and half of those who are overweight are considered obese. As a result, weight loss is an important priority for many people. Even so, it isn't an easy process, and it is often difficult to gauge success initially. In short, losing weight can feel like an uphill battle.

Most people who are overweight have already tried to lose weight, time and time again. Sometimes they find temporary success, but they often end up gaining that weight back in the long run.

A huge market of weight loss products, supplements, and programs exist to service those wanting to lose weight. Even though it sounds cynical, the truth is that the weight loss industry capitalizes on the heartbreak and desperation people often feel about their bodies. And many are willing to pay for a weight loss solution; the U.S. weight loss market totaled $64 billion in 2014.[1]

Turn on your TV or look in any magazine, and you'll find advertisements for all sorts of weight loss supplements. Or you'll see that one device that you have to use for only five minutes a day that gives you perfectly toned abs (sure).

The message is enticing but ultimately misleading. Exercise is really not a five-minute endeavor, and any pill that promises to dramatically shed pounds will be ineffective at best and could even be dangerous, as many of these pills have not been reviewed by the FDA. If any one of these pills or fast fixes is the "magic bullet" for weight loss, then why are so many people still unsuccessful in their efforts to lose weight?

Most people *can* lose weight. However, keep in mind that obesity is usually the result of a series of bad decisions. People don't become obese overnight, and losing that weight is going to take a proportionate time and effort commitment. Don't waste your time or money on gimmicks.

Some have argued that you can be "fat and fit," and to some degree this statement is true. Even at an increased body weight, having good habits like regular exercise and eating fruits and vegetables can help improve your health. However, carrying excess body weight not only puts increased stress on our joints and tissues, but also is metabolically harmful, increasing the risk of many diseases and health problems in the future.

Unfortunately, there is no shortcut to successful—and sustained—weight loss. It comes from making better food choices and getting in more movement. And truthfully, it can't be one or the other. You cannot out-exercise a bad diet. And on the other hand, you cannot lose weight simply by counting calories while being a couch potato. Long-term weight loss comes from both eating better *and* getting more exercise.

Here's another important point to remember as you go: Weight loss is different for everyone. Just because a girlfriend of yours dropped 15 pounds in two months doesn't mean that you necessarily will. (And don't forget that people who lose weight quickly sometimes gain it back just as quickly.) Conversely, you may encounter people who have struggled for years to lose a couple pounds, to no avail. Don't compare yourself to others. Every-*body* is different and your experience will be unique to your own metabolism, diet, and activity level.

Finally, I hope you will make a commitment right now to embrace your body no matter what shape it is in. It is perfectly okay to love yourself despite needing (and trying) to get healthier. It is better for your mind, body, and soul to nurture yourself even while you push yourself to make better decisions. The weight loss experience I encourage is not a masochistic boot camp, and I don't encourage you to use shame or self-imposed cruelty as a motivational tool on your journey. Your entire experience of regaining your heart health and vitality can and should be one of affirmation and even joy. Remember this as we move forward and start making heart-healthy new habits.

How to Approach a Major Lifestyle Change

As we've discussed, change is hard for everyone. It takes us out of the comfort zone of our usual (and often bad) habits. Yet, once we start eating better, we eventually come to crave those foods that are healthier for us. And once we start exercising regularly, we can feel that familiar waning of energy after a few days of not doing so. The good news is we *can* "reset our compass" to desire better foods. We might still enjoy a piece of pizza or a bowl of ice cream on occasion, but for the most part we'll be able to satisfy ourselves with healthier choices, like a big salad or a hearty bean chili.

Dean Ornish has said, "Joy of living is sustainable; fear of dying is not." Changing our lifestyle because we fear having another heart attack is sustainable only for a very short period of time. Eventually, that fear of danger wanes, and our bad habits are likely to creep back in. Positive, rather than negative, reinforcement is necessary for permanent change. When we have more energy, feel better about ourselves, and are generally happier, we will be able to better sustain our positive lifestyle choices.

When we decide to overhaul our bad habits, there are two ways to approach things. We can choose, as Harold did, to make changes all at once. Or, we can choose to do things one step at a time. For example, that can mean starting with eating better— cutting out fast food, eating meals at home, and incorporating more fruits and vegetables. The next step may be starting to walk for exercise. And once the exercise is a solid habit, the next step may be to do even better with the diet—adopting a plant-based diet. Either approach can work. From my own personal journey, I know that I took things one step at a time to get to my own current healthy habits.

In this book, I will show you the habits that are best for your heart. The more of these habits you can take on, the better your health will be. Yet even small changes can bring about results. Merely going from a completely sedentary lifestyle to walking five or ten minutes a day will lead to improvements in health. But, since you're reading this book, you're likely more motivated to make greater changes. And remember that with more major positive diet and lifestyle changes, you can really be your best.

Truly embracing change takes time: anywhere from 30 to 90 days. It can take time to get accustomed to new foods, new eating habits, and to moving more frequently. It may feel strange not to have a piece of meat on your plate, or to need to eat more vegetables. Walking 30 minutes may initially feel tiring or even impossible. When you eat more fruits and vegetables and legumes, you may feel gassy as your digestive system becomes accustomed to dealing with more fiber. These are short-term discomforts that must be overcome to achieve long-term health benefits.

And when we try to change, sometimes we stumble. It's all part of the process. As you approach making any major changes, it's wise to expect a few delays and pitfalls. Keep trying and you will eventually succeed. To give you perspective: Smokers who try to quit often aren't successful on their first try; in fact, it takes an average of eight to eleven attempts at quitting before most smokers are successful. However, with each subsequent attempt at quitting, your likelihood of quitting gets better.[2]

Tips for Success as You Change Your Habits

Everyone is different. Just as there are many different body types and different personalities, there are many different tactics and "tricks" for making changes stick. You may or may not need to try all of my suggestions below—however, I have found that these yield good results for most people.

Get to the (psychological) root of your habits. Various psychological issues can contribute to our eating habits and lifestyle choices. Do you snack on chips when bored or stressed? Many times people turn to food (or television marathons) as ways to tune out or self-soothe. And in extreme cases, people use food or unhealthy behaviors to cope with past traumas such as abuse. A therapist can help you recognize these tendencies and deal with the underlying causes. She might also be a good resource to help you mentally to make changes and visualize your success.

Be accountable. Accountability is key to making positive changes. Programs such as Weight Watchers, where you have to weigh in and keep track of points for various foods, can increase your chances of success. Technology can help with accountability too. An online food tracker like MyFitnessPal lets you record your food and water consumption, and keeps track of how often you exercise. Apps like this will make you think twice before you reach for a cookie.

Seek out social support. This goes hand in hand with accountability. Often, people who work out with a buddy or join a group do better at making and maintaining change than those lone wolves who try to power through on their own. For instance, you might join a heart health support group or meetup to exchange recipes and also to share your victories and frustrations with others who face the same issues. Or you might get involved in a Zumba class or a hiking group—working together with like-minded people can be incredibly empowering and can make what might otherwise seem like drudgery feel like actual *fun*.

Make your home a healthy zone. Allow no junk food in the house and stay stocked up on good, nutrient-dense foods. If unhealthy foods are in reach, it is too easy to reach for one small treat and slip back into bad habits. If you are hungry enough, you will eat the healthy food in your home and find that it satisfies you after all.

Get the rest that you need. For most people, adequate rest consists of 7-9 hours of sleep per night. When you are deprived of sleep, you are more likely to make poor food choices and less likely to exercise. Establish a routine in which you go to bed and wake up around the same time most days. Also remember that it's even more important to get plenty of rest when you are forming new habits that require energy and a clear mind. Sleep enough to ensure that you feel rested when you wake up.

Plan for success. Plan out the meals you will eat for the week ahead of time. Make a list before you grocery shop and stick to that list. Also, know in advance if you will be dining out, and plan on eating extra-healthy during the time leading up to that meal. (Restaurant food often tends to be higher in calories than the foods you would prepare at home.)

Plan your exercise as well. Just as you wouldn't skip an important meeting or abruptly cancel on a date, don't skip out on your workouts! Think about exercise as an "appointment" on your calendar. As a matter of fact, actually pencil in workout time in your planner. This makes you more likely to actually go to the gym or go out for that jog.

Hire some help. If you can afford it, you can use additional resources to help you achieve your health goals. Work with a personal trainer. This is someone who not only gives you appropriate exercises to help you reach your goals, but provides another layer of accountability! Or—if cooking isn't convenient—perhaps you can pay someone to batch cook and freeze a few meals for you. (Though later on, I'm going to share with you how to easily and quickly prepare meals for yourself.)

Don't assume that these kinds of services are only for the wealthy. Even people of modest means can hire a relative or neighbor to help out with the cooking. Or you might "barter" with a trainer or someone who already does a lot of cooking: "In exchange for giving me some training tips, I'll do your taxes," or, "If you'll prepare three meals a week for me, I'll give your daughter piano lessons." With the right motivation and a bit of creativity, you can come up with some great solutions.

Consider going on a retreat. Going away to a safe place to make changes can be a dramatic turning point in your life and empower your new choices. TrueNorth Health Center in Santa Rosa, California, is one such place. There, one can be evaluated by a team of medical professionals, enjoy healthy plant-based meals, learn to prepare those meals upon returning home, exercise, and practice yoga. For more information, visit their website at www.healthpromoting.com.

Reward yourself when you meet a goal. Treat yourself to a massage, a new outfit, or simply an afternoon with that new book you haven't had time to read. Some people may reward themselves based on number of pounds lost, but I don't recommend that. (Remember, weight loss is not the goal; getting healthy is.) Rather, consider rewarding yourself when you make it through, say, two weeks of sticking to your exercise routine. And when you hit a big milestone like, say, six months or a year, pamper yourself with something "bigger" like a weekend getaway.

Here is one final success tip: *Take it a day at a time.* Don't expect a magical overnight transformation. Changing your lifestyle for the better is definitely a marathon instead of a sprint. If you have a bad day and backslide a little, accept it and move on. Don't wallow on the setback and don't use a small slipup (or two) to justify more bad decisions. Get up and keep trying. This is a major key to sticking with any type of change…over time, you *will* start to see (and feel) results.

SECTION II

Exercise Made Easy

A Brief History of My Fitness Journey (and What You Can Learn from It)

Some people think the "fitness gene" is something you either have or you don't. This is a total misconception. Yes, some people may be slightly more predisposed toward athletics, but I want to dispel the myth that anybody's fitness potential is predetermined or some sort of natural gift. I've seen too many people wholly transform their bodies and health to believe that for some it just can't be done.

Take me, for example. I was an ordinary person who became an endurance athlete by practicing and working hard. While you certainly don't need to start doing triathlons in order to be healthy, it should encourage you to know that no matter where you're starting from, you can improve your fitness. And if you have cardiovascular disease, it greatly benefits you to get into better shape right now. You *can* defeat heart disease, the same way a runner gets through a tough race: one determined step at a time. In the next chapter, I'll share how you can get started incorporating exercise into your daily life. But first, let me tell you a little about my journey to becoming an athlete.

I don't have an extraordinary fitness background. In fact, in kindergarten, my inability to balance on my right foot landed me in "special gym" for kids who were felt not to have much athletic aptitude. Still, I did participate in some fitness activities in my early life. I played soccer in the local youth leagues, and ran cross country up until age 11, when a fractured leg from a tobogganing accident sidelined me for the next couple of years.

A couple years later I took up cheerleading because my high school had a sports requirement, and I enjoyed performing with my squad in front of the crowd during games. I also spent a couple seasons on the junior varsity softball team—though admittedly, I wasn't very good, and spent most of my time on the bench learning to juggle softballs.

While I maintained a normal weight as a child and teenager without any worry, I was not so lucky when I left for college. I was a vegetarian at the time, and dorm life included a dining room without a lot of good vegetarian choices, and ample pizza and soft-serve ice cream available at every meal. Even though the drinking age was 21, alcohol was everywhere and a big part of social life. I consumed more than enough calories from the flavored punch of the moment at fraternity parties, or on weeknights out at bars that never carded anyone. And once the bars close, what is good to eat? Pizza!

In addition to my questionable freshman diet, I didn't exercise regularly. In my first semester of college, I gained 20 pounds, and in the second semester piled on another 7; I started college at 5' 9 1/2" and 145 pounds and 10 months later weighed in at 172!

After gaining so much weight, I decided to take action. I realized that I would be starting medical school soon and knew that as a doctor I would be telling my patients to eat right and exercise, so perhaps I needed to start setting a better example for them. And so I got off my butt and started making one small fitness change at a time.

First, I started rollerblading everywhere I went. In the gym I began lifting weights and did mind-numbing cardiovascular exercises on whichever machine struck my fancy. I also took some measures to improve my diet, including preparing many of my own meals at home. As a result of all this, I dropped a few pounds and began to look and feel better overall.

Then, in my third year of medical school, I started running. While I didn't realize it at the time, this new undertaking would prove to dramatically shape my entire life. At first I could barely run more than a mile or two. But, as I persevered, I would go three or even four miles at a time. I signed up for a 5k race, finishing proudly in a time of 31 minutes. Soon I could run five miles routinely. Looking back, I can see that I crossed a threshold during this time: Exercise stopped being an effort and started becoming a priority for me—a seamless part of my life.

In 2000, I signed up for my first marathon, the Chicago Marathon, as part of the Leukemia & Lymphoma Society's Team In Training, an organization that coaches participants to complete an athletic endurance event while raising funds for research and patient care. Raising $2,500 proved harder than training my body to run 26 miles, though both goals were tough.

Training was challenging at times, because I worked up to 80-hour weeks as an internal medicine resident with occasional overnight hospital shifts. I recall doing one 16-mile run after having spent the past 32 hours inside the hospital! I finished that marathon in 5:37, which is a respectable time, though since then I have completed marathons significantly quicker. One year later, in 2001, I ran the Detroit Free Press Marathon in a slightly faster time of 5:15.

Thereafter, my endurance athletics ambitions temporarily lessened. I finished my internal medicine residency, got married, and moved to Rochester, New York, for my cardiology fellowship. I continued to eat a fairly processed lacto-ovo-vegetarian diet and yo-yoed 15 pounds one way or the other, depending on how well I was keeping away from junk food and nighttime snacking. I continued to run for exercise, maybe two to four miles at a time, and eventually started working out regularly with a personal trainer.

Fitness wise, all seemed well…until, at age 28, I developed a nagging pain in my right foot. After multiple X-rays, bone scans, and MRIs, I was diagnosed with tendinitis. I would wear an orthopedic boot intermittently, get excited when I felt there was improvement, start running again, and then the pain would return. The cycle continued until I bought a good pair of running shoes with custom-made orthotics and was patient enough to wait until I could safely run. Unfortunately, this was 16 months of my life in which I was unable to run.

While healing from this injury, I found other ways to be active. I started bicycling with an old piece-of-junk mountain bike I had sitting in the garage. I joined a women's cycling group out of our local bike shop and eventually purchased a new road bike. I took up swimming as well and joined a local masters swim group. I spent most of my time in the slow lane, but during that time I learned to bilateral breathe during freestyle and gained some swim endurance.

Between swimming and biking, my injured foot was able to heal. I had finally started listening to my body. Now armed with new running shoes and custom orthotics, I could gradually ease back into running. But, at this point, I was really enjoying mixing up my training, and thought a bit about maybe doing a triathlon.

My spinning instructor, Mary Eggers, was a triathlon coach, and I asked her if she could coach me to be ready for a sprint triathlon in three months. She helped me prepare for the sprint distance Finger Lakes Triathlon, a 0.45-mile swim, 13-mile bike ride, and 3.1-mile run. My training schedule consisted of six days of workouts, totaling about 8 hours per week. Intense though this schedule was for a cardiology fellow in training, I managed to do most of the workouts.

I started to swim in open water in addition to my pool swimming. Canandaigua Lake near Rochester was quiet, peaceful, and a great place for practice swims. My group had weekly open water swims, and I practiced swimming in my wetsuit and swimming without relying on the walls of the pool to push off.

Race day came, four days after my 30th birthday. I did well and had a great time! My swim was a few minutes faster than I had expected, the bike portion went okay, and I had far more energy for my three-mile run than I anticipated. My father and my husband came to cheer me on, and they along with my triathlon friends really motivated me to have a great day.

These were the "peaks" of my life but, like everyone else, I also went through some valleys. A few months after the triathlon I just described, my husband and I decided to divorce, after only two and a half years of marriage. We didn't part bitterly, but any ending like that is hard, and for me it led to some fear of my future. I already knew I had an upcoming one-year interventional cardiology fellowship position at Tufts Medical Center in Boston—an incredibly competitive placement—and while excited for this opportunity, I was afraid of what my future held on my own. And, at this low point in my life, I was hurt and trying to heal.

What better way to pour out my emotions than through training? So, throughout the winter of 2006, I swam, I biked, and I ran. Actually, I mostly ran, because it made me feel best. I could run out my anger and my loneliness. I had a personal trainer, and I had told him of my goal to run faster. He gave me special workouts for the treadmill and soon I saw my running pace pick up.

After a few weeks, I could consistently complete a single mile in under 10 minutes, and one day a few weeks later, I was excited as I ran a sub-9 minute mile. That spring, I ran my fastest 5k race yet, the Fairport 5k, in 28:14, at just over nine minutes per mile. Later that summer, I completed five triathlons, two in Upstate New York and three near Boston.

In my last race of the summer, the Hale Off-Road Kidz2Camp Triathlon, I placed first out of the four women in my age group. It was a small fundraising race, and I think a lot of the participants were parents of kids going to that camp, but still, as a newbie to the sport of triathlon, first place certainly feels nice!

As I completed my interventional cardiology fellowship in the spring of 2007, which would be my seventh and final year of training before working as an attending cardiologist, I contemplated where to move. My divorce was finalized and I didn't need to worry about moving with someone, so I could go anywhere in the country. I chose Los Angeles. Not only would I have family there, but I would have amazing weather to swim, bike, and run outdoors year-round.

At the end of the summer of 2007, I completed my first Olympic-distance triathlon, the Los Angeles Triathlon, a race that started with a swim at Venice Beach, followed by a bicycle ride across the city of Los Angeles into downtown, and a two-loop run through downtown Los Angeles. Later that fall, I ran the City of Angels Half Marathon, and in the spring of 2008 the Los Angeles Marathon, my first marathon in seven years, faster than both previous marathons.

I aimed for bigger and better races and decided that it was time to step up my game and sign up for a half-Ironman distance race, which is made up of a 1.2-mile swim, 56-mile bike, and 13.1-mile run. In order to prepare properly and give my best performance for the 2008 season, I decided to hire a coach, Jamie Silber.

Under his instruction, I competed in triathlons, including the aforementioned half-Ironman, and several marathons, along with some smaller races. I bought a fancy bike designed for triathlon racing, and I continued to exceed my personal bests as I continued training. The process wasn't always easy. Even though I loved training and racing, I faced stops and starts along the way, and periods of burnout, when I didn't feel like training. I even ran one marathon wearing a Supergirl costume to remind myself not to take it all too seriously.

The following year, 2010, my main goal was the daunting Ironman™ with a 2.4-mile swim, 112-mile bike, and 26.2-mile run. This race is the "Mt. Everest" for many endurance athletes. I opted for Ironman Lake Placid, a race in Upstate New York, because I had spent so much of my time there between school and rotations. I knew I'd come across Mary Eggers, my first triathlon coach, whose guidance got me across my first triathlon finish line five years earlier.

Ironman training was more time-consuming than anything I had done up until that point. Getting ready to complete a race of that distance required some long bike rides that were longer than anything I had ever completed. As the bike was my weakness, Coach Jamie assigned me several long bike rides for training.

I can recall my longest ride of 125 miles. I started in Santa Monica, met a friend a few miles later in Pacific Palisades, continued along the Pacific Coast Highway to Malibu, where I met a group of triathletes at Zuma Beach, then continued with them out past the Point Mugu Naval Base. Then my friend Lee rode with me all the way out to Oxnard, until we turned around and came back. She finished up at Zuma Beach, and I rode the entire distance on my own back to Santa Monica, exhausted at the end. The training was often tedious, but I kept in mind that it was necessary in order to complete an Ironman.

The race itself was exhilarating. There's nothing like standing with 2,600 other athletes, hearing the gun go off, and the commotion of limbs thrashing in the water. I got kicked in the chin within 30 seconds, and numerous elbows to the side, but five minutes in, the crowd thinned enough such that I was able to get into my groove and swim well for the 2.4 miles. I saw my parents and a few friends cheering me on as I got onto the bike. The 112-mile bike ride was indescribably beautiful as I sailed through the Adirondacks.

I felt suffused with energy as I ran the 26.2-mile marathon, and kept a slow but consistent pace for the first six miles—and then my right knee started aching. The pain worsened, and while I was able to maintain a shuffle of a run, it was almost excruciating. I put on my best grin as I crossed the finish line and heard the announcer yell out, "Heather Shenkman, you are an Ironman!" What an incredible feeling! Despite the pain in my knee, and really my whole body, I can honestly say this was one of the peak experiences of my life—in that glorious moment, all the hard work, agony, and exhaustion was worth it.

While I was thrilled to have earned the title of "Ironman," my knee was sore for weeks later. I swore that I was "one and done" and that this would be my only Ironman distance race. I did not need to put myself through that training or pain again. I could call myself an Ironman and that's all I needed.

During this time I joined the Fortius Racing Team, which was coached by Gerardo Barrios. I ran more marathons, triathlons, half-Ironman distance races, and even my first ultramarathon, a 50-kilometer (31 mile) race—each time beating my previous record.

One of my greatest and most interesting challenges came in 2013, at the Maccabiah Games in Israel. It is the third largest sporting gathering in the world, with nearly 10,000 Jewish and Israeli athletes of all ages from over 70 countries coming together to compete. This was my first opportunity to compete internationally as a triathlete. In addition, I had the chance to compete in four different events occurring over the course of eight days in the "Maccabi Man and Woman" competition: a 26-kilometer bike ride, a half marathon, an Olympic distance triathlon, and a 5-kilometer open water swim. The heat hovered around

100 degrees, but I hung in there and, of all the women ages 35 and up who completed the four events of the Maccabi Man and Woman competition, I placed third, earning a bronze medal.

Five years after my first Ironman race, I decided to take on the Ironman distance again. (So much for my "one and done" proclamation!) As I saw dozens of my friends bragging about having signed up for Ironman Boulder for 2015, I too took the plunge. Perhaps it was a bit of peer pressure, but truthfully, somewhere in the back of my mind I was wondering, *Can I beat my previous Ironman time?* And this time I was part of a team that would be competing—including Coach Gerardo—so I knew that the race would be a whole lot of fun, and the training would be more interesting.

I'm so glad I competed. My second Ironman experience ended up far better than my first. The training was less monotonous, with dozens of triathlon friends racing, and on race day, I had an exhilarating time! In fact, I finished over an hour faster than my first attempt at the Ironman distance five years earlier!

That brings us to today. I've described to you my journey from non-athlete, to casual runner, to Ironman triathlete. As my story shows, I certainly didn't become an Ironman overnight. It was an evolution that started long ago and still continues today. Between trying to lose a few pounds in college and aiming to set a better example for my patients, I discovered a passion that I didn't realize I had, and it has vastly shaped my life.

My goal in writing this book is not to turn you into an ultra-endurance athlete. Rather, I want to show you what I have done and convince you that you can achieve more than you believe. I started from a point of almost zero fitness and never dreamed that

I would someday compete in some of the most rigorous races on earth.

If you are reading this book, chances are that you or someone you love is suffering due to a heart-related illness. I've shared my story because I want to encourage you simply to try. Try something small now to improve your health, because small efforts lead to bigger efforts, which lead to even bigger efforts—and eventually they start to pay off.

You will experience valleys, hills, plateaus, and even mountaintops on your journey to better health. You'll have days when you feel stalled-out and don't want to commit yourself, followed by breakthroughs that make you feel like you're on top of the world. Those victories are the moments that matter, and when they happen, you will be glad you worked so hard to achieve them. But it all begins by taking one small step that will then lead to another.

I promise you are capable of making a fitness transformation that will make you feel better than you may have thought possible. In the pages ahead, I will talk about the benefits of exercise and describe how you can incorporate healthy and safe movement into your routine so that you give your heart the support it needs to be strong and vital.

No matter where you start from, you can channel your inner athlete and move more. I will show you the way. With time and effort, you can become more active and ultimately improve your health, your fitness, and even your mood! Let's head toward the "starting line" together.

CHAPTER 5

Fitness and You: Why You Should Exercise

Staying active is important for our health and well-being. Historically, humankind's survival has been dependent upon the ability to move. Whether running away from wild animals, foraging for food in the forests, caring for and wrangling children, or building shelter from the elements, people long ago had plenty of opportunities to get daily exercise and movement.

However, modern life has changed all of that. Our basic needs for survival are much easier to come by than they were hundreds of years ago, and we no longer have to move in order to stay alive. Plus, we have modern time-consumers to contend with, such as long work hours and plentiful TV and Internet distractions. In fact, we no longer need to go to the store—at the touch of a button on our smartphone, we can buy groceries and order necessities that we otherwise would have had to venture out to a store to purchase. Now that we have all the luxuries of modern life, are we better off being sedentary just because we *can* be? Of course not!

Our bodies perform their best when we get plenty of physical activity. But for most of us, the low-intensity movement of our daily lives is simply not sufficient to achieve ideal wellness. Unless you are a valet who is running to get cars, or a bicycle delivery person, or a mail carrier who walks several miles a day for his or her route (and maybe not even then!), you need daily exercise.

Because this is a book about heart health, I am going to focus mostly on the health benefits of cardiovascular exercise. "Cardio," or cardiovascular exercise, consists of continuous movement, maintaining an elevated heart rate for a sustained period of time and burning calories. The whole purpose of cardio is to exercise the heart muscle—which is beneficial to each person, but especially those at risk for or suffering from heart disease. While weight training and stretching are certainly valuable for increasing flexibility and building bone strength and muscle tone, when it comes to maintaining heart health, cardiovascular exercise is irreplaceable.

Why You Should Make Exercise Part of Your Life

Everyone knows that they "should" exercise—we see sports drinks advertisements glorifying athletes, and apparel companies spend fortunes to glamorize fitness. And by now, everyone knows someone whose life transformed when they discovered CrossFit or SoulCycle. Yes, exercise is an industry, so there's no shortage of people telling you to get active. But, glitzy marketing aside, it's important to remember the reasons *why* everyone needs to work out.

There are many legitimate benefits to exercise. Even if you aren't looking forward to adopting a fitness habit, these arguments for working out should help convince you to do what's best for your body. Exercise is known to reduce the risk of heart attacks and stroke, lower blood pressure, control and prevent diabetes, fight osteoporosis, and reduce the risk of several kinds of cancer. It is also helpful for stabilizing and treating other illnesses such as fibromyalgia and chronic lung disease. Additionally, exercise keeps the mind sharp as we get older and helps to combat dementia. The message is clear: If you want to enjoy great health, it pays to start exercising right now.

But that's not all. Exercise does more than just keep your body healthy—it also supports a healthy mind and spirit. Maybe you've heard about the connection between mental health and exercise. If not, let me fill you in. Exercise fights depression. When you work out, your body creates hormones called endorphins. Endorphins trigger a positive feeling in the body and they are responsible for the pleasure you feel when you enjoy a piece of chocolate, watch a funny movie, or listen to a song you love. Likewise, whenever you work out, these magical chemicals create a feeling of happiness and well-being. Finally, exercise is good natural medicine for managing the stressors of everyday life. Just try it after a tough day (instead of curling up with a bowl of ice cream or crawling into bed for a nap). Going for a run or bicycle ride is the perfect way to blow off steam or literally "work out" feelings of anxiety and worry. I always return from a workout feeling happy, invigorated, and ready to tackle anything that comes my way.

And let's not forget that, in addition to its many health and wellness benefits, exercise helps you look great. When you exercise, your skin glows, you lose excess weight (which we also know is important for total heart health), and you are able to witness your body becoming sleeker, well-defined, and more capable.

The bottom line is this: There is no reason *not* to exercise and every reason *to* exercise—especially when you realize that your general health is already less than optimal simply by being sedentary.

How Much Exercise Is Enough?

Hopefully by now, you are ready to hit the gym, the hiking trails, or the bike paths to get active. But you may be wondering, *Well, how often should I be exercising?* The American Heart Association recommends the following for overall cardiovascular health:

At least 30 minutes of moderate-intensity aerobic activity at least five days per week for a total of 150 minutes

OR

At least 25 minutes of vigorous aerobic activity at least three days per week for a total of 75 minutes; or a combination of moderate- and vigorous-intensity aerobic activity

AND

Moderate- to high-intensity muscle-strengthening activity at least two days per week for additional health benefits.

However, for those looking to lower blood pressure and cholesterol, the AHA recommendation is an average of 40 minutes of moderate-to-vigorous physical activity at least three to four times per week.[1]

Although you may need to start slower if you are coming from an extremely sedentary lifestyle, you should try to work your way up to the point at which you can reach these recommended goals. You can get there if you dedicate yourself to this goal. Start small if you need to and realize that any exercise is better than none at all.

On a practical level, I recommend my patients perform 30 minutes of exercise five days per week. Believe me, this is an achievable goal. You can find at least 30 minutes out of your day to dedicate to your health. But, for improved fitness, I encourage more exercise, perhaps aiming for up to an hour of exercise five times a week.

How Intensely Should I Be Exercising?

IMPORTANT: BEFORE YOU START ANY EXERCISE PROGRAM, YOU SHOULD DISCUSS YOUR PLAN WITH YOUR DOCTOR. While I am a physician, I am not your physician and do not know the details of your health. I will discuss

general guidelines for starting an exercise program, but until you get the go-ahead from your doctor, do not start exercising.

Remember that the purpose of cardio is to exercise your heart and lungs, so if your idea of a workout is taking a slow and easy walk, know that you probably aren't achieving the optimal level of intensity for benefitting your heart. Generally speaking, most exercise should be done at a moderate aerobic level. This means that you are breathing hard. I encourage patients to use the "talk test" to figure out if they are working out hard enough. Imagine someone is exercising next to you. You should be able to have a conversation with him or her while you work out, but it should not be easy to talk due to breathing harder.

In addition to achieving a moderate level of aerobic activity, I also encourage my patients to incorporate bouts of more vigorous exercise during some of their workouts. For example, if walking, incorporate some hills or add in a few jogs. If going out for a run is more your speed—pun intended—try adding some light sprints to your routine. The point is to achieve a baseline level of cardio and then gently stretch that threshold. These more intense intervals can help to build stamina and endurance as you train. You'll notice that during these periods of time, the "talk test" might be more challenging; perhaps you're just able to get out a few words at a time due to breathlessness. When first challenging yourself with these bursts of intensity, remember to take them slow and steady as you gain stamina—at no point should you feel severely winded, lightheaded, or dizzy.

Tips for Sticking with Exercise

For some reason, the hardest part of exercise is getting started. Often it is challenging just to take that first step out the door to go for a walk or jump in the swimming pool. Many people have a mental block about exercising, and as a result they resist and procrastinate indefinitely. My advice for this universal problem is: "Don't stop to think about it; just get moving." Put on your sneakers and workout clothes and head out the door. As soon as you are actually going for that brisk walk, or warming up in your fitness class, you'll realize how simple and effortless exercise really is, and you'll no longer feel dread about it.

But, once you get started, you have to stick to your fitness routine in order for it

STAY SAFE! Always Remember These Rules:

- Ask your doctor before you start exercising.
- Stop if you feel dizzy or lightheaded.
- Warm up and cool down before and after exercise.
- Don't push yourself too hard.
- Drink plenty of fluids before, during, and after exercise.

75

THE VEGAN HEART DOCTOR'S GUIDE

to be effective. Here are a few tips to help you stay committed and enthusiastic about working out:

Find partners. Who says working out has to be a solitary chore? I like to use my exercise time to be social. It's great fun to work out in a group setting or even with just a friend. When I'm exercising with a group, I can use the energy of the others working out around me to encourage myself to do my best. Also consider joining a social media exercise group to build camaraderie and keep you motivated and accountable. Apps such as MapMyRide or Strava allow you to upload your workouts and share them with your friends, allowing for some friendly competition.

Change up your routine. Doing the same thing over and over *can* be boring. That's much of why I love triathlon. There are three different sports—swimming, bicycling, and running—that keep me engaged both during training and throughout the race. Beyond those three sports, I like to mix up my training with an occasional boot camp class, spinning, or yoga. You can mix up your fitness in the same way. Maybe do a fun cardio class for a few months and then switch to something new. And feel free to change things up according to the seasons. During the spring and summer, aim to do plenty of outdoor activities so you can take advantage of the nice weather.

Find something you enjoy. If it feels like a chore, you're not going to stick with it. So figure out what you like and avoid workouts that aren't fun for you. Personally, I do not love being on a piece of equipment at a gym. But everyone is different, and I am confident you can find a way to exercise that you love and even look forward to! So if you enjoy spending 30 minutes on an elliptical at the gym, by all means do it. If you love to dance, go out dancing or take a Zumba class. If you love nature and the outdoors, go for a hike.

Reward yourself. Adopting a fitness routine that you can stick with is tough work, so you can use rewards to incentivize and reinforce healthy exercise patterns. Remember that we are wired to seek pleasure, so the promise of a small reward can help you get up and move when you would rather relax. If you know that you need a little motivation to get moving, create a personal incentive plan and give yourself a small reward after you reach an exercise goal. For instance, after walking for 30 minutes, reward yourself by taking a hot bath or reading a magazine you enjoy. When you are able to jog a mile without stopping, buy yourself something special to celebrate and to help you associate exercise with pleasure.

Now that I've told you all about the great benefits of exercise and shown you ways to make it an enjoyable experience, I hope you are inspired to lace up your shoes and go for a walk. I totally believe you can do it, and I am counting on you to do what's right for your heart and your overall health. In the next chapter, we'll talk more about different types of exercise and how they are each beneficial.

CHAPTER 6

Get in Motion: An Overview of Different Types of Exercise

By now you know that exercise is crucial for your health, and not just for your heart health. Exercise helps to keep you energetic, maintain a healthy weight, elevate your mood, and keep your brain healthy as you age. I believe that exercise should be a joyous part of your day every day—or at least five times a week.

Before we explore what types of exercise might benefit you the most, I want to address just how important the lifestyle shift you are about to make truly will be. Becoming active through exercise—combined with the changes you are making to your diet—is paramount for your health, but it is also an overwhelmingly important aspect of your very humanity.

Here's what I mean by that: Exercise is so much more than a change that you tack on to your existing routine. It is a paradigm shift that will crack open the status quo and transform your life. To make this change, not only must you change what you do each day, but you must change how you think about life itself. As I've stated before, we are not meant to be sedentary creatures but healthy, strong, ever-moving ones. Physical exercise is inherent to being human, but many trappings of modern society work against this natural plan. While our ancestors (and even our great-grandparents) lived continuously active lives and connected with nature, we now think it's normal to sit at a desk all day on our butts, and to drive home from work and then sit on our butts in front of the TV all night. But nothing could be further from normal.

However, changing the entrenched sedentary patterns that got you to your current state of health is not easy. For this reason, the *form* of exercise you choose *must* be compelling to you. It has the job of breaking you out of the mindset that your old way of life is "okay" and "normal." By finding a form of exercise you feel passionate about—like I did—it becomes much easier to change your life. And while you may not *always* feel super eager to lace up your walking shoes and bound out the door, exercise should never be a dreaded chore. That's the old mindset stubbornly trying to pull you back to bad health—don't give in to it!

In this chapter, we will talk about various types of exercise you can choose from. Remember that some exercises may be more strenuous than others, so as you select and settle into your exercise rhythms, you should be mindful that you're adequately giving your heart a healthy workout. And, as there are several types of exercise to choose from, you may want to incorporate a few different varieties of exercise into your weekly routine. In fact, I strongly encourage this. Not only will mixing up your workouts keep things interesting, but it will continue to challenge your endurance and your muscles in different ways.

Now let's talk about what types of exercise you might want to do!

Walking

Walking is the simplest form of exercise you can get. All you need is a good pair of walking shoes and somewhere to walk—whether that is a neighborhood, a mall, a track, or a treadmill. And if you are sedentary or otherwise start- ing out with exercise, walking is an excellent form of move- ment—especially if you find yourself struggling to get in motion. As with all forms of exercise, start slowly and lis- ten to your body.

As you become accus- tomed to walking, find ways to challenge yourself. If you are walking outdoors, find routes that have some hills or carry hand weights to give you some additional resis- tance. If you are on a tread- mill, play with the speed and the incline until you find a

A Word on Walking in Nature

As I have mentioned, much of modern life is spent quarantined from nature. We live, work, and, in many cases, even play indoors, and many of us rarely come into contact with the natural world. But I believe that spending time outdoors drastically improves our lives. Feeling sunlight on your face, the wind on your skin, or a spray of ocean water harmoniously connects you to your humanity and makes you feel great. So while heading to the gym is a fantastic choice, try to spend some of your ex- ercise time doing something outdoors too. Whether you walk or jog along a nature trail or go kayaking on a river, you'll benefit from the nature all around you and experience a deeper sense of peace. You might also consider joining an outdoor fitness group to get your nature fix and meet new people.

setting that pushes you a bit. In the mall, perhaps add a couple of flights of stairs to your walk.

My 92-year-old grandmother walked on the treadmill nearly every day at her senior apartment, up until just before she passed away, and her commitment to staying fit even as a senior inspires me every day. She prided herself on her "pupils," other seniors who lived in her apartment building, who would join her for her 30-minute walks. Her regular walking and remaining active helped keep her far more able-bodied than others her age.

Running

Running is my passion, and it just might become yours too. If I have a short period of time and need to get in a workout, I'll go for a run.

Why should you choose running for *your* workout? Like walking, it's easy and inexpensive—all you need is workout clothing and a pair of shoes. Further, like walking, running is a convenient form of exercise. There's no need to "go" anywhere to start my workout, all I need to do is head out my front door. (Though, to change it up, I do enjoy running along trails or in the park.) Finally, for me, I feel like running is therapy—I get the best endorphin rush, also referred to as a "runner's high," after a good run.

Running isn't for everyone, of course, and that is fine. You should always find a workout that resonates with you. That said, if you are a walker and want to start running, it's best to ease into running by adding short running or jogging intervals to your walks. For example, you may start with one minute of jogging followed by five minutes of walking, and continue building upon that pattern. As you get fitter, you can lengthen out the jogging intervals and shorten the walking intervals, until your workout is entirely a jog!

Water Workouts: Jump in the Pool!

I hear far too often from my patients that they cannot exercise thanks to their back, their knees, their sciatica, and so on and so forth. Luckily I have a great solution for these types of impediments: Get in the pool! Water provides natural resistance for your muscles while it also lessens impact to your joints or other problematic areas.

There are plenty of ways to get a workout in the water. Swim laps on your own or with a masters swim group. Take an aqua aerobics class. Or, just get in the pool and move! For me, swimming laps with a masters swim group is a fun challenge and a great way to be social and exercise, especially on a hot summer day. Swimming is a great recovery workout as well; if I've just had a long run or a bike ride, nothing feels better than getting in the water; taking some long, slow strokes; or kicking with a kickboard to loosen up my legs. No matter what your fitness level, you can benefit from using a swimming pool as part of your fitness regimen.

Bicycling

There's no better way to take in beautiful scenery and get in a good workout than by going for a bike ride. Make sure your bicycle is in good repair, that your tires are well pumped, and of course that you are wearing a helmet. (I may have cautioned a patient or two that I did not work hard to open their coronary arteries just to have them crack their head on the pavement.)

Look for bicycle paths or trails local to you and local cycling groups that ride at your ability level. Here in the Los Angeles area, we have Griffith Park, the Los Angeles River Path, the Rose Bowl, the Santa Monica Mountains, and many other great areas that I've had the chance to explore on my bike.

If you want to ride indoors, find spinning or group cycling classes at your gym. I love a class with good music and an enthusiastic instructor to guide me through a challenging workout. I'm less enthusiastic about solo stationary bicycle riding, as it is far too easy to set the bike at a low resistance speed and to mindlessly spin your legs without working up any sweat at all. If you do choose to ride a stationary bicycle, make an energetic playlist with upbeat music that will encourage you to challenge yourself.

Group Exercise Classes

Nothing pumps me up like being with a group of people who are working out—the energy in the room is palpable and contagious. While aerobics may have been the craze of the '80s, and Tae Bo classes a relic of the '90s, there are so many great group workout classes that you can find at a gym. If you love to dance, there's Zumba or even a traditional dance class like jazz or ballet. You can get a great burn in a boot camp-style or high-intensity interval training class. Or, there are group weightlifting classes if you want to tone and sculpt while getting an aerobic workout. One of my favorite group exercise classes is at a freestanding gym called Barry's Bootcamp. It's an hour-long class with 30 minutes of treadmill intervals and 30 minutes of strength training with body weight and weights.

Yoga

Yoga is based on a Hindu practice that encompasses breath control, meditation, and the adoption of specific bodily postures. Today it is practiced all over the world for health and relaxation. There are many types of yoga. The yoga that most people think of is hatha yoga, which is the movement through several postures and breathing techniques. There are more challenging yoga classes that may call for handstands and more advanced poses, and more low-key classes such as restorative yoga, which involves relaxing poses that are held for up to five minutes at a time.

There are many health benefits to practicing yoga. While it may not necessarily build up your endurance or fitness level, yoga is great for stretching, balance, and relaxation. And it also has notable health benefits. Yoga has been demonstrated to lower blood pressure. One small study of 57 subjects demonstrated a drop of six points in the systolic blood pressure over the course of 12 weeks of either once or twice-weekly yoga classes.[1] Yoga can also effectively treat depression and anxiety; it is thought that yoga affects the stress response, leading to improved mood.[2]

If you decide to try yoga, it's best to begin with a group class or private instruction—and not a video. In a class, an experienced instructor can teach you to properly execute the various positions you'll see over and over throughout your practice.

Strength Training

For cardiovascular health, your top priority should be aerobic exercise, or exercise that will raise your heart rate. However, if you choose to make the time, strength training can be beneficial for maintaining strong bones as we get older, keeping balance, and for looking and feeling toned and fit.

As the name implies, strength training involves using resistance to work out and, well, get stronger. You don't need to lift heavy weights to get the most out of your strength training sessions, but you should lift a weight that challenges you. In fact, you don't even need weights; exercises such as squats, lunges, push-ups, and dips challenge you while using your own body weight for resistance.

If you are new to strength training, it may be useful to schedule a few sessions with a personal trainer who can observe your form and suggest some exercises that are best suited to you. Further, strength training can be done in a class setting, as described earlier. I've found that strength training complements my training, and I incorporate it a couple of times a week into my own regimen.

I've given you some ideas of different ways that you can exercise. Now it's time for you to begin. I encourage you to explore, to try new ways of exercising, and to find things that you enjoy doing so that fitness feels less like a chore and more like an enjoyable part of your routine of life.

CHAPTER 7

Finding the Energy, Motivation, and Discipline to Exercise

We have finally reached the place where the rubber (of our collective sneakers) meets the road. Hopefully by now you have an idea of what a manageable fitness routine might look like for you—or at least you are willing to try a new class, or see what it feels like to go for a walk or a light jog after work. I applaud your determination and willingness to venture into intimidating new territory with me.

You may be wondering how you will manage to make such a drastic change to your life, especially if you have been sedentary for a long time. I believe manageable, lasting change comes down to a combination of motivation, energy, and discipline.

This chapter is dedicated to giving you some practical and effective tips for sticking with exercise so it can become a regular part of your life.

First, let's talk about motivation. It's especially important to motivate yourself when you're just starting out and exercise is "new." Being excited about and engaged in your exercise routine will make the experience that much more enjoyable than approaching fitness with dread or annoyance. You can combat any fear or anxiety you're feeling—and thus drastically increase your motivation level—by trying out the *Exercise Motivators* I've listed. These tips will ease your transition into physical activity and help you look forward to your daily workouts.

Next up, we have the energy factor. Maybe you feel motivated to work out, but your life is so hectic and stressful that you can't imagine taking on an extra responsibility. In addition to reminding you that exercise creates a *very* powerful boost in your energy levels, I'd like to add that when you realize the stress-reducing benefits of exercise, you'll have no problem fueling yourself properly in order to make it through a workout. Take a look at the section titled *Exercise Energizers* to learn how to prepare your body and mind for the physical and emotional requirements of a workout.

Finally we come to discipline, which is probably a loaded word for many people. Nonetheless, discipline is an important factor in sticking with exercise. Don't be dismayed if you are not a naturally disciplined person. I believe that when you structure your life in a way that makes exercise practical, accessible, and fun, you have already tapped into a disciplined approach to exercise. The tips in this chapter, combined with the other instructions in this book, will help you achieve that discipline organically—as a by-product of your preparation, enthusiasm, and energy. Consult the tips found under the heading *Fitting Fitness In* to learn how to structure your life in a way that supports your choice to work out regularly.

Now, are you ready to move? Great! Here we go.

Exercise Motivators

Buy workout clothes you'll look forward to wearing. No one wants to work out in ancient, worn out sneakers with old pajama bottoms and a ratty t-shirt. Invest in a few nice pieces so you will feel put-together and confident as you begin this new routine.

Keep in mind that workout gear does not need to be expensive, but it *should* be comfortable. For men, find comfortable elastic shorts or pants and a t-shirt or tank. For women, go with leggings, loose pants, or shorts for bottoms and a t-shirt or tank for your top. Ladies, be sure to invest in a supportive sports bra; sports bras are better than standard bras because they are sweat-wicking and more supportive for activity. In fact, pick all of your workout fabrics carefully. I generally advise against cotton workout gear because it holds in sweat and moisture, whereas technical synthetic fabrics are sweat-wicking and lighter weight.

Finally, don't bother blowing the bank on expensive workout wear, unless you just want to—no judgment! You can find durable, stylish athletic clothing brands at every price point, so I recommend buying some good inexpensive basics to get you started. You can always expand on your workout wardrobe as you progress.

Get a gadget. You may find a fitness tracker to be motivating in your fitness routine. Sometimes it's nice to know how many steps you took in a day, how far you walked this week, or how close you are to walking the distance of the coast of California. Fitness trackers are great at helping you put your daily movement into perspective.

Some fitness trackers have GPS, the ability to monitor your heart rate, measure your sleep, and other fancy features, but a basic device that counts your steps could be all you need. It does not need to be expensive! My father wears a Fitbit every day. He will not go to bed until he completes his 10,000 daily steps. Whenever he visits, he often will walk laps in my driveway until he gets to his full 10,000!

Pick your playlist. Music helps you get in the zone for a workout and will inspire you along the way. Set the tone for a great workout with upbeat tunes you love. It can be fun to intentionally create your workout playlist, and then to add to it whenever you find a great new tune. Fill it with up-tempo songs that motivate and encourage you. My playlist, which I call "Music That Makes Me RUN," is mostly electronic music, hip-hop, and top 40, but also includes the Rocky theme, "Gonna Fly Now."

Get your just rewards. There's nothing wrong with rewarding yourself for a workout well done. Changing your lifestyle is no easy feat, and working toward a goal—and a reward—will give you something to look forward to while building good, healthy habits. So set a reasonable yet challenging fitness goal to strive for, and when you reach it, treat yourself with something that will make you smile.

Now this isn't permission to buy yourself a present every single time you hit the gym. You're trying to develop discipline and create healthy fitness habits, and those don't happen overnight. Therefore, it's important to set a goal that you'll have to work to achieve. For example, your goal might be to work out at least every other day for a month. This is a challenging yet reasonable amount of time, which pays off in many ways. When you complete your month of workouts, not only will you have a well-deserved reward, but you will also be that much closer to solidifying your budding fitness habit, which will serve you for the rest of your life.

Need some ideas of great rewards that won't derail your progress? Try some new workout gear. Or maybe you'd like a deep tissue massage to help ease sore muscles. You could also have a facial or a similarly pampering spa treatment. You've worked hard and deserve to celebrate!

Have a backup plan. Don't let a cold or rainy day keep you from working out. Be ready with a backup video workout or some home exercises you can fall back on.

Here's another good backup plan: Go to the mall and join the leagues of mall walkers there. I remind my patients, when they complain about the weather (Yes, they complain about the weather in Southern California! I'm from Detroit; I don't quite get it.), "Your heart doesn't care what the weather is like outside." Treat your heart right and find a way to get the workout in.

When I'm in a crunch, like when traveling, and I want to find a good workout, I'll go to YouTube and punch in keywords like "quick cardio workout" or "strength training." There's a lot of free short videos available on the internet so you have plenty of options and no excuses. There are also streaming fitness channels available on cable or Roku/Apple TV, so keep all these resources in mind the next time it's raining or freezing outside.

Exercise Energizers

Stay properly hydrated. You have probably already heard how essential good hydration is to your health. When you've had enough water, you feel fuller, more energetic, and your body will work better. The idea is to get enough water all the time, not just before or during your workouts.

So throughout the day, drink water whenever you're thirsty. If you get bored with plain water, jazz it up by adding some lemon wedges or frozen fruit to your glass. And remember that liquids found in watery vegetables and soups help hydrate you as well.

If you're planning to be working out in the heat, or if you know you're going for a longer workout, plan to hydrate extra and bring water with you to drink while you exercise.

Fuel up before and after your workouts. You shouldn't go into a workout when you're overly full, but having a light snack before hitting the gym or the trail will give you the energy to get through your workout. We will go further into addressing healthy snack options later in the book, but for now, focus on eating a pre-workout snack that is easily digestible and not too heavy.

Before my morning workouts, I will drink a homemade soy latte and eat a banana with almond butter. Or sometimes I enjoy a fruit and vegetable smoothie for energy and hydration. After your workout, have another light snack, or if it's close to your regular mealtime, just enjoy your next meal.

Get enough rest. To experience boundless energy throughout the day, pay attention to how much sleep you're getting at night. Sleep is necessary for peak performance. If, for some reason, I haven't gotten good rest (such as when I'm called in to the hospital for an emergency at 3:00 a.m.), I usually skip my morning workout, and either get in a shorter, easier workout later on, or I just count the day as a "rest day." Aim to get between seven and nine hours of good sleep every night. Your body will thank you, and you'll notice that you will have the stamina to get the exercise you need.

Make relaxation time a priority. Don't become so committed to the changes you're making for your health that you forget to schedule some downtime. If you overschedule your days to the point that you're constantly exhausted, you won't feel like exercising regularly. So build in some relaxation to bring balance back to your life.

Choose relaxing pastimes that you enjoy. Indulge in a midafternoon nap, take a bath, or zone out with a TV show you love (but don't go crazy and spend the whole night on the couch). And, for ultimate relaxation, get a massage! It helps keep your muscles and tissues healthy, reduces risk of injury, and just feels great.

Fitting Fitness In (Sneaky Techniques for Sticking with Exercise)

Pencil in your workouts. When you treat exercise like any other scheduled event in your life, you're more likely to stick to it. So put your weekly exercise schedule on your calendar the same way you would remind yourself to go to the grocery store or show up for an important meeting. Keep it somewhere you can see it, like on your fridge, and when you complete each work out, be sure to check it off and enjoy the sense of accomplishment you feel.

Make exercise a family affair. It can be tricky to make room for exercise when you have children (or other family members) to care for. But being responsible for your kids' well-being doesn't have to prevent you from achieving your fitness goals.

Find activities you can do with your kids or spouse, so together you can all become healthier. Hold a weekend family volleyball tournament, take a long hike together, or just a family walk around the park. When you teach your kids about fitness early on, you are helping them form healthy habits now, which will set them up for better health down the road.

Combine your work life with your workouts. Chances are, your job is a major part of your life. But your dedication to work doesn't have to prevent you from staying fit or active. In fact, you can find ways to merge your work life with your fitness routine. Here are some ideas to get you started:

- Walk to your lunch destination. If you usually head to a nearby café for lunch, consider walking there. Or take the second half of your lunch break to go on a short walk. Remember, cumulative movement adds up over time, so every step you take counts.

- Form a walking club with colleagues. You and your coworkers can meet a couple times a week before or after work to walk a quick mile or two. This is a good opportunity to enjoy the social benefits of group exercise.

- Does your place of work have a gym? If so, take the opportunity to melt away work-related stress while you melt off those extra pounds.

- If you live close to work, consider a walking commute when the weather is nice. Or consider biking. But do this only if there are clearly marked sidewalks or bike lanes along your route.

- Try out a standing desk part-time. If your work environment allows, use a standing desk some or all of the time to reduce the amount of time you spend sitting down. If you're not able to stand up to work, at least be sure to get up and move around a bit once an hour.

Take the road less traveled. Bonus movement counts when you're trying to transform from a sedentary lifestyle to one of movement and fitness. So go the extra mile (literally) by working a few extra steps into your day any time you are able. To do this, take the stairs whenever you have the chance. This is a great way to sneak in a few extra minutes of exercise. I make it a rule to avoid elevators as much as possible. Whenever you go shopping or to any sort of appointment, be sure to park at the back of the parking lot and take a brisk walk to your destination. And if you live in a bustling city, try to walk—not drive—to nearby cafés, stores, and appointments whenever possible.

Optimize quality time with friends. Instead of meeting friends for a beer or for dinner, meet for a walking date or a drop-in fitness class like yoga or barre. Not only will exercising together enhance your friendship bond, but you will be supporting each other's health in a meaningful way.

Exercise when it makes sense for you. Are you a morning, evening, or afternoon person? The answer probably indicates the best (and worst!) times for you to work out. I'm definitely a morning person. I function so much better during the day when I have done my morning workout. I evolved to become a morning person during my interventional cardiology fellowship, because the day could go very long and evening workout plans could easily be derailed. But, most of the time, barring emergencies, I knew that my morning was my own, and that is when I would exercise.

Over time, I just grew to be someone who enjoyed that pattern to the day.

Don't fight against your natural energy rhythms or lifestyle rhythms—*work* with them! Do you absolutely know that you won't wake up 30 minutes early to walk before work? No problem; just exercise when it feels good to you, maybe in the afternoon or even at night. A 9:00 p.m. jog can be just as satisfying and productive as a 9:00 a.m. jog. Just be sure to wear reflective gear so you are visible after dark.

Hopefully this advice has made your fitness forecast seem positive and possible! In conclusion, let me remind you that the most useful tip in helping you make exercise an integral part of your life is to adopt the right attitude about the many changes you are making for your health. Remember this: It is helpful to view exercise—along with your overall commitment to wellness—as a marathon, not a sprint.

This attitude will help you maintain perspective and gain renewed motivation when you slip off track (and you likely *will* slip off track from time to time; it happens). Don't create unrealistic expectations about working out every single day, no matter what. Life happens, and you may not always be able to stick to an iron-clad workout regimen.

That said, remember that you are on a continuous journey to better fitness and that means committing to your health and body every day. If you do slack off for a week, or fall off your diet, which we will be discussing in the next section, don't let guilt or a sense of shame mire you down. Remind yourself that you are on a quest to live as healthily as possible, that the journey is just as important as the destination, and that you are absolutely worth the effort it all takes.

Embracing a Plant-Based Diet

My Dietary Evolution: How I Made the Journey from Eating Animals to Eating Plants

My journey to embrace a plant-based diet was a gradual process that spanned many years. I grew up in a home where meat was served with dinner every night, and chicken nuggets and Happy Meals were frequent treats. I had a brief awareness, as most kids do, around age eight or nine, that these meals of animal foods were made from a former living being. That phase didn't last long, and I went back to eating animals without much thought.

My brother was the first to become a vegetarian in our family, which was due to an ethical decision he made at ten years old after seeing chicken wings "dissected" in science class. He did everything he could do to convince the rest of our family to go vegetarian as well—from joining PETA to making sure that there was always some piece of animal rights literature lying around to making obnoxious comments when we would eat meat.

A few years later, as he was preparing for his bar mitzvah, he told my parents he refused to wear *tefillin*, the leather straps that are a traditional part of the ceremony. My father made him a deal: If my brother wore the *tefillin* during the ceremony, then my father would become a vegetarian for one year. They both followed through with their deal, and, extraordinarily, my father has remained a vegetarian ever since.

Around that same time, at the age of 16, I sympathized more with the plight of animals, and I decided to become a vegetarian as well. I had read enough and seen and heard enough from my brother to be aware that animals suffer terribly. Thinking about this subject was deeply upsetting to me, and one day I just couldn't bear the thought of eating another animal. Soon after, with no meat in the house, my mother followed our example and gave up meat as well. Since then, my entire immediate family has been vegetarian.

My first few weeks as a vegetarian were tough. Giving up my Taco Bell chicken soft tacos and Chinese restaurant orange chicken challenged me to find new options for dining out. At this point, I was still eating a lot of fast food and restaurant food, so instead of my old meat-themed choices, I frequented Taco Bell for bean burritos, and I found that vegetable lo mein or a tofu stir-fry were good options for Chinese restaurants.

I remained a vegetarian through college, though that vegetarian diet wasn't necessarily the healthiest. As I have previously mentioned, during my freshman year in college, I gained 27 pounds by eating too much pizza, ice cream, fast food, and late night eating.

And, even though I was a vegetarian, I didn't eat that many vegetables initially. It wasn't until a date night at an Indian restaurant that I realized just how tasty vegetables could be, and from then on I started incorporating more of them into my diet. During medical school I cleaned up my eating a bit, by preparing more meals in my apartment and eating more vegetables.

I continued making gradual improvements to my eating habits, but as a first-year internal medicine resident, I still had my vices. When on call overnight, I would run around the hospital with a 20-oz. bottle of Coke, and would guzzle it all by the end of the evening to keep me awake and alert. The Little Caesars outlet in the lobby of Henry Ford Hospital, open late at night even after the cafeteria closed, tempted me always, for a late night slice of pizza or crazy bread.

While I initially became vegetarian because of my love of animals and disdain for their cruel lives and painful slaughter, I realized more and more that a vegetarian diet was a *healthier* choice as well. And then I realized that it wasn't a vegetarian diet that was the key, but rather making whole-food, plant-based, or as some would say, vegan, choices, and that dairy and eggs were not necessarily healthy choices.

When I started my cardiology fellowship training, I started to think seriously about a vegan diet for myself. I had picked up a "Compassion Over Killing" pamphlet at a local restaurant, which truly made me think more about the plight of farm animals and that the dairy and eggs I was consuming also came from horrific cruelty. In addition, I was reading about the work that Drs. Esselstyn and Ornish had done to successfully reverse heart disease with a plant-based diet.

It took me over a year from that initial spark of insight to finally decide to take the leap from lacto-ovo vegetarianism to becoming vegan. To put it mildly, Rochester, New York, where I was living at the time, and where I was completing my general cardiology fellowship training, was not the most vegan-friendly city. There, even a vegetarian diet seemed radical to most. What would it be like to be a vegan? *Would I go hungry?*

I still remember the first day I decided I would be vegan. I was working late at the hospital, and I recall roaming the cafeteria for something to eat that was vegan. Salads weren't a big part of my repertoire at that time, so the salad bar didn't really appeal. I ended up making myself a peanut butter and jelly sandwich.

However, with the support of monthly potluck meetings of the Rochester Area Vegan Society, my transition to veganism became easier. I learned all sorts of ways to prepare healthy vegan meals that were appealing, interesting, and delicious. And, being surrounded by other vegans, I felt less like an outcast.

That was 13 years ago. Since then, I've moved to Los Angeles, a more veg-friendly city, and as time has passed, plant-based diets have become much more mainstream than they once were. Now there are plenty of plant-based restaurants, and just about any restaurant is able to prepare a good vegan meal. And, high-quality plant-based products abound in grocery stores today, from a variety of non-dairy milks to different varieties of tofu and grains. And because it's fine to enjoy the occasional dessert or treat on special occasions, you can find an impressive and tasty selection of vegan cookies, brownies, and non-dairy ice creams in markets everywhere. But remember, although vegan sweets are truly amazing, they are "sometimes" foods, and do not replace a healthy diet full of vegetables, fruits, and whole grains.

My own diet has evolved further from "vegan" to more "plant-based." When I first decided to be vegan, I didn't eat that many vegetables or salads, and I ate a lot of the "fake meat" foods that many people try to live on once they go vegan. A salad was hardly a meal to me; after all, how could something sitting on a bed of lettuce actually be filling? Luckily today, my grocery shopping trips are less in the middle of the store where the processed food is kept, and more at the periphery of the store, where the fresh produce can be found. Also, I take a weekly trip to the local farmers market to purchase the locally grown fruits and vegetables that are the staple of my diet.

I chose to move at my own pace, as we all do when making big changes that will improve our lives. However, I encourage you to learn from the experiences I've shared as you launch your own transformation. I promise that you can find great satisfaction without compromising food quality in a plant-based diet. You don't have to subsist on questionable "frankenfoods" to try and trick your body into thinking it's eating meat. Nor do you have to live on carrots and lettuce. Instead you can enjoy whole healthy foods that make you feel so satisfied you don't miss the meat in the first place, like overflowing wraps stuffed with roasted veggies, savory stews loaded with flavor, and even a delicious slice of pizza now and then!

Here's the bottom line: Changing my diet changed my life and my health. Plant-based diets are proven to prevent and even reverse heart disease. They can change your life too, but only if you commit to them.

In the next section of this book, I am going to show you how to begin your own transition to a plant-based diet. First, I will share the ethical, environmental, and health arguments for giving up meat and animal products. Then together, we will cover plenty of tips and tricks to help you adopt a plant-based diet with ease, and we will also learn some fun delicious recipes so you have plenty of tasty food options and never have to miss out on fun or flavor! I hope you are hungry to learn…now let's get cooking!

CHAPTER 8

The Case for a Plant-Based Diet

Making a drastic change to your diet is a pretty big step. It requires adopting a new set of practices, learning intimidating new skills for some (cooking!), and a commitment to spending time outside of your dietary comfort zone. But it is a step that is worth taking and has the potential to change your life for the better. The right diet can really turn your health around.

If your eating habits are like most people's, you doubtless already know that a change is in order—possibly, a *big* change. If you eat fast food at least once a week, if you guzzle sodas each day, or if a significant portion of your food comes from a box, a package, or a wrapper—you definitely need to transform your diet. And if you are already suffering from a heart condition or are at risk for stroke, then a dramatic change to your eating habits is an absolute must.

I personally follow a vegan diet, or what I prefer to refer to as a whole-food, plant-based diet, and I advocate for my patients to do the same. I know that asking you to give up your beloved meat, dairy, and eggs is a tall order. But switching to a plant-based diet is very doable, and in fact can be delicious. Before I tempt you too much by appealing to your appetite, let me first lay out the reasons why a vegan diet is so very important. When you understand why it's better to eat this way, it is easier to change.

In this chapter, I hope to make the case to you that a plant-based diet is not only the best diet for your health, but is the kindest way of eating for animals and for our planet.

My initial motivation to follow a vegan diet came from my compassion for animals. The more I learned about how animals and animal products come to our table, the painful lives they lead and terrible deaths that they suffer, the more I knew that I did not want to contribute to this horrific cruelty. But, as my training as a physician continued, it also became apparent that eating plant-based foods prevented and treated many of the diseases that so many of my patients were facing.

Unfortunately, very few people realize the value of a plant-based diet and they are reluctant to change. Most of us are raised believing that animal products are necessary parts of our diet. To some, nothing is more American than a hearty breakfast of bacon and eggs, or a dinner of steak and a baked potato complete with butter and sour cream. Often my patients tell me that they eat animal products because they grew up eating them, and this seems "normal." And, yet these are the foods that lead to the diseases I treat every day.

Unfortunately, vegans suffer from an (unfounded) image problem. We are often viewed as being on the "fringe"—overly idealistic, pleasure-impoverished hippies who subsist on lettuce and are scrawny and weak from lack of protein. Nothing could be further from the truth, of course. Some of the world's best athletes, from gold medal Olympian Carl Lewis, ultramarathon champion Scott Jurek, professional triathlete Hillary Biscay, NFL players David Carter (also known as "The 300-Pound Vegan") and Griff Whalen, mixed martial arts fighter Mac Danzig, and champion bodybuilder Patrik Baboumian, among others, follow plant-based diets. Further, a plant-based diet has fueled my own success as a triathlete.

Another problem is that many people today are uneducated about good nutrition. We learn our "facts" from what we see on television and online. And that information is very much influenced by the meat and dairy industry, which spends millions of dollars promoting their products. Unfortunately, there is no powerful lobbying group to promote the health benefits of spinach and kale. Further, the 2015 Dietary Guidelines for Americans was heavily influenced by the meat and dairy industries, and as a result, the general public receives very biased information about nutrition.

Most doctors don't talk much, if at all, about nutrition with their patients. And there are many reasons why. First, doctors' schedules are busier than ever; when you have only 15 minutes with a patient, it is hard to squeeze in time for a discussion of diet—there are too many other pressing matters that also need attention.

Another barrier to doctors' discussing nutrition is a blatant lack of knowledge. It is unfortunate, but doctors don't necessarily know much about nutrition, because as medical students they themselves didn't learn much about the subject.

I graduated from Albany Medical College in 1999; at that time, my school was one of the few that had a nutrition curriculum. That curriculum consisted of a total of 16 hours over the course of the first two years of medical school, which is not much compared to the many hours of pathology, pharmacology, anatomy, biochemistry, and other subjects that took up our time, but was more than what was offered by most other medical schools.

The nutrition information that we did learn didn't focus on issues that relate to common problems we see today in America. The majority of the curriculum consisted of learning about conditions of malnutrition that would be encountered mainly in third-world countries. An example is kwashiorkor, a severe form of protein malnutrition associated with edema and skin rashes, and marasmus, which is severe malnutrition of babies and children.

While these conditions are indeed horrific and demanded study, they didn't necessarily apply to the majority of the people we students would be treating in *this* country. And although it would have been extremely helpful, we didn't learn about the consequences of the typical high-fat, high-sugar, highly processed diet that most people in modern countries follow. Although, through my work, I see the consequences of this diet play out every day in my patients.

It is ironic that in one of the richest countries in the world, nutrition is one of the major causes of disease. Fast food, packaged snacks, and sodas from vending machines are all too easily accessible and affordable, while healthier foods, like fruits and vegetables, are much less readily available. And, these poor diet choices are major contributors to the three major causes of death: heart disease, cancer, and stroke.

So, if what we eat is so important for our health, then why don't future doctors learn about nutrition? While this is speculation on my part, my feeling is that nutrition may not be perceived as scientific, and therefore is not sophisticated enough to be taught. Yet the *effects* of people's diets *are* measurable in a scientific manner. We have, at our disposal, all the published statistics on heart disease, and there is actual evidence of its treatment through dietary and lifestyle changes.

It is a terrible shame that food, a vital foundation of life, is mostly overlooked in medical schools—especially now that we understand the correlation between diet and health! The standard American diet is making people sick on a massive scale, yet there is little initiative to educate people on how their dietary choices affect their health. I would like to see this change in the future.

Finally, some food choices are deeply ingrained in our culture (think giant billboards promoting soft drinks and fast food joint commercials that bombard us with tempting close-ups of fries), and people are widely perceived as being unwilling to change their eating habits. From my own experience, I believe this not to be true. Patients can be very motivated to learn and make changes if it improves their health.

That said, if your doctor doesn't know a lot about nutrition, and isn't advising you about what you should be eating for your health, that doesn't mean that you can't learn about nutrition and make good food choices for yourself. Much of what I know and what I counsel my patients on about food and nutrition comes from what I have learned and read on my own. In fact, in order to expand my own knowledge of nutrition science, I took a

Do Your Own Research

Take charge of your health the proactive way! Here is a list of websites that I refer patients to. These provide excellent guidance on nutrition and health in general:

www.nutritionfacts.org

www.nutritionmd.org

www.pcrm.org

www.nomeatathlete.com

I urge you to spend some time exploring these resources as you seek to learn more about how to fuel your journey toward better health.

comprehensive online course through Cornell University and earned a certificate in plant-based nutrition from the T. Colin Campbell Center for Nutrition Studies. There is a wealth of information out there that you can utilize to improve your health.

Now, I want to share the arguments for a plant-based diet with you here so you can see just how effective, humane, and environmentally conscious this way of eating can be.

For the Animals

I am a cardiologist, and the argument for a plant-based diet from the perspective of health is strong on its own. However, I think it is important to know exactly where your food came from. If you watched the process of how your meat, fish, eggs, or cheese got to your plate, it is unlikely that you would want to eat it.

Over time, our population has grown; hence our consumption of animal products has increased. As a result, the small family farms that once produced our meat, eggs, and cheese have been replaced by large corporate factory farms. Animals are now treated as commodities and objects, confined to large warehouses, in crowded cages, pens, or stalls for most of their existence.

Birds raised for their meat—chickens and turkeys—are confined to such densely populated sheds that the ammonia from their waste causes painful burns to their skin, eyes, and respiratory tracts. To keep the birds from pecking one another in such cramped conditions, about one-third to one-half of the length of their beaks are cauterized without anesthesia, leaving these birds in severe pain for weeks.[1]

Egg-laying hens are crammed into even smaller spaces, so small that many hens die of dehydration or asphyxiation. Dead corpses are often found on the floors of the cages. The battery cages that the hens are placed in are so small that they can't even spread their wings.[2]

Pregnant pigs live in gestation crates so narrow that they cannot even turn around, and are forced to lie on uncomfortable metal grates. Piglets are separated from their mothers after just a few weeks. Their tails are chopped off, the ends of their teeth snipped with pliers, and the males are castrated, all without painkillers. Pigs are naturally very clean animals who avoid soiling their living areas, and yet they must spend their lives in crowded pens on concrete slabs in dark warehouses. This denies them from practicing their natural behaviors like lying in the sun, playing, and using their keen sense of smell to explore.[3]

Dairy cows are repeatedly impregnated via artificial insemination. Yet it is very rare that a dairy cow nurses her own babies.

Of the male offspring, some are sent to slaughter immediately, while others are tethered to small stalls and confined to crates for their short 16- to 20-month lives, at which point they are slaughtered to become veal. Once the dairy cow is no longer productive, she too is slaughtered for her meat.[4]

What about fish? Though they perhaps seem less personable than larger animals, fish have a response to pain that is similar to mammals and birds. In fact, fish are intelligent enough to learn to avoid fishing nets by watching other fish in their group and can also recognize their "shoal mates." Upon capture, these fish are often crushed, impaled, suffocated, and gutted while fully conscious.

Nearly half of all fish consumed in the United States are raised in "farms," which are crowded and dirty. As a result, many fish suffer from infections, diseases, and injuries. Those fish that do survive are starved for days before transport to slaughter, in order to decrease contamination of the water during transport. And, the process of catching fish in the wild with large nets leads to the killing of "nontarget" animals such as sharks, birds, sea turtles, seals, and whales that also get caught in the nets. Furthermore, fish in the food supply often have high quantities of mercury and PCBs, which are harmful to humans.[5]

For the Environment

Production of animal products for human consumption vastly contributes to the destruction of our environment. You may be surprised to know that the leading source of greenhouse gases is not automobiles, but rather comes from the factory farming of animals and animal products for food. Cows, for instance, release methane into the atmosphere through their frequent "emissions."

Additionally, livestock consumes large quantities of water and contaminates our water supply with their waste products, antibiotics and hormones, chemicals, and sediments from eroded pastures. Further, raising animals on land has led to deforestation, particularly in Latin America and the Amazon rainforests.

Conventional fishing also has a large impact on the environment. Overfishing can reduce the overall sustainability of an ocean environment, affecting the marine population levels and impacting the food chain of a region. This ultimately has led to the extinction of some species. Coral reefs have also been destroyed by overfishing—both by destroying the coral with nets and by reducing the fish populations that keep the underwater algae balance in check. Bottom trawling, or running a net along the ocean floor, destroys a large amount of sea life—basically anything in the path of the heavy, giant nets. And "by-catch," or unintended animals caught in nets, may be killed in the process.

Fishing farms also harm their surrounding environment, as waste products such as uneaten food, feces, and dead fish contaminate the local water supply, along with the pesticides and veterinary drugs that are fed to the farmed fish.

For Our Health

While there are compelling reasons to eat plant-based for the animals and for our environment, I focus in my daily work on preventing and treating heart disease. It's good to know that eating in a way that is good for the animals and the planet is also optimal for your health! For me, the connection between a plant-based diet and good health is all too clear—as I treat patients who have lost their health at least partially due to their poor dietary choices.

In the words of Hippocrates, "Let food be thy medicine and medicine be thy food." To this day his guidance rings true—food can be medicine or food can be poison. What we choose to eat has a huge impact on our health.

Plant-based diets are associated with a lower risk of many diseases, including coronary artery disease, diabetes, hypertension, obesity, osteoarthritis, and several types of cancer. In fact, populations who follow predominantly plant-based diets live longer than most.

"Blue Zones" are five geographic areas identified as having the greatest longevity. These five Blue Zones are Okinawa, Japan; Loma Linda, California; Nicoya Peninsula, Costa Rica; Icaria, Greece; and Sardinia, Italy. The five areas have the following traits in common: a high priority of family, low rates of smoking, mostly vegetarian diets (with the exception of Sardinia), moderate physical activity, and frequent consumption of legumes.

The Seventh-Day Adventist Church, for example, urges its followers to embrace a "well-balanced vegetarian diet." The Adventist Health Studies have found that those following vegetarian diets live significantly longer than non-vegetarians.[6]

Findings like these seem to be compelling evidence that diet may be a factor in living a long life. While I certainly advocate that my patients also get adequate exercise, avoid smoking, and develop rich, full social lives, I am most concerned with their diets. I have seen my own patients reverse their heart disease by following a plant-based diet. Furthermore, not one of my patients who has adopted a plant-based diet has suffered another heart attack or even required another stent. That is evidence enough for me.

How a Plant-Based Diet Benefits Your Heart

Plant-based diets provide huge benefits to the heart in partic-ular. Dean Ornish's studies from the early 1990s were some of the first to look at plant-based diets and heart disease. Patients with coronary artery disease were randomly divided into two groups. The patients in the control group received standard care and were given the traditional recommendations of a "low-fat diet" and reg-ular exercise. The experimental group, on the other hand, received instruction on eating a healthy, mostly plant-based diet (partici-pants were permitted a small quantity of low-fat dairy), along with exercise, meditation, and group support.

After one year, the experimental group's heart health looked much better. There was a 91 percent decrease in angina or heart-re-lated chest pain, huge drops in cholesterol, and 82 percent of pa-tients in this experimental group had a decrease in the amount of plaque in their arteries.[7] Keep in mind, it is typical for many, if not most, patients to experience coronary disease progression, and for arteries to become *more* clogged over time. So it is very impressive that these patients demonstrated reversal of plaque build-up. Even after five years, patients following Ornish's lifestyle program con-tinued to have a decrease in the amount of plaque in their arteries.

On the other hand, those in the control group continued to experience worsening of their disease. In fact, they had more than twice as many cardiac events, such as heart attacks or the need for angioplasty or surgery, as patients in the experimental group.[8]

Doctor Esselstyn's Groundbreaking Experiment

Dr. Caldwell Esselstyn, a surgeon at the Cleveland Clinic, had a strong family history of coronary disease. His own father had his first heart attack at the age of 43 and had cholesterol levels as high as 300. Dr. Esselstyn took pride in his work in treating disease with surgery. Still, he wanted to primarily focus on how to prevent disease in the first place.

In the late 1980s, Dr. Esselstyn found 24 patients with end-stage coronary artery disease, a group he described as "a sorry lot by the time they arrived in my office—sorry in terms of both their physical health and their spirits." They had prior open-heart surgeries, angioplasties, stents, had frequent angina chest pain, and were on numerous heart medications. His ambitious goal with this group of sick patients was to arrest and reverse their coronary disease through diet.

He put all of these patients on a diet free of animal products, oil, or nuts, permitting only a small amount of fat-free milk or yogurt. The patients received thorough instructions on diet and were followed at frequent intervals to help them stay compliant with the diet. They received standard medications, which in some patients included cholesterol-lowering statins—these were just becoming part of the standard of care in the 1990s for heart disease.

Of the 24 patients who started in the study, 18 were able to stick with the diet for a total of five years. All six who were unable to follow the diet had cardiac events, from needing stents or bypass to having heart attacks. On the other hand, none of the 18 who followed the diet had an event during that time, and many outlived the predictions of their physicians. Images taken of the heart support this success as well—coronary angiograms were performed on some of these patients before and after the diet, demonstrating the reversal of even critically severe blockages of coronary arteries. Nuclear stress test images also show dramatically improved blood flow to affected parts of the heart.[9]

Years later, Dr. Esselstyn looked at a larger group of patients.[10] This study, published in 2014, in a modern era of treating heart disease, followed 198 patients with disease of the arteries. The patients received similar intense counseling on a plant-based diet free of nuts, oils, and seeds. Of those who started, 89 percent were able to stick to the diet over the course of an average of 3.7 years. Those patients who stuck to the diet had a much lower cardiovascular event rate of 2.3 percent, compared to a 52 percent event rate among those who could not follow the diet. Further, angina chest pain improved in most patients following a plant-based diet, while the chest pain of the others actually worsened in most.

Now that I have given you many good reasons to follow a plant-based diet, I hope that you are eager to embrace it. This diet is good for the animals, good for the environment, and great for your health. And I understand that you may be nervous about the difficulty of adopting a new way of eating. Don't worry. With a little guidance, it's really not a hard transition to make. We'll talk later in the book about how you can transition to, and thrive on, a plant-based diet.

CHAPTER 9

Eating Plants: How to Go Vegan Without Going Out of Your Mind

Here you are, ready to take yet another important step that will change your life and your health forever. You have now made the decision to adopt a plant-based diet and supercharge your nutrition to lose weight, prevent or reverse cardiovascular disease, and safeguard yourself from stroke and diabetes. Rest assured, the effort you put into adopting your new way of eating will pay off for the rest of your longer, stronger, healthier, and happier life.

But before we jump in, here is another success story about one of my patients who overcame the odds—not only by surviving a major cardiac event, but also because she drastically changed her diet and is now thriving.

When Nancy was only 48 years old, she developed an unusual pain in her chest during her aerobics class. An ambulance was called and she was quickly rushed to the hospital where doctors discovered she was having a heart attack. Luckily Nancy survived, and decided right then to start following a plant-based diet. She got to work seeking out tasty vegan recipes and discovering healthy ways to incorporate whole, plant-based foods into her diet. Before long, her new dietary choices became habit and she never looked back. Since then, Nancy has done remarkably well. She still exercises regularly—in fact, probably even more intensely than before—and thanks to her healthier food choices, she has lost and kept off about 15 pounds since her heart attack.

Nancy is a prime example of someone who turned their life around after a serious health crisis. Instead of defeating her, Nancy's heart attack *empowered* her to make healthier food choices. And her subsequent weight loss gave Nancy the confidence as well as the ability to get even more fit and further improve her health. Keep Nancy's progress in mind as you learn all about transitioning to a plant-based diet. You can become a success story too, and I will show you how starting right now.

Let's begin by addressing what is sure to be your biggest concern: At first glance, transitioning to a plant-based diet seems overwhelming (maybe even impossible). I understand how you feel! You are essentially overhauling eating habits that you've developed over a lifetime. It's normal to feel hesitant or outright afraid. Relax. These simple steps will set you up for success and help you view each day as an opportunity to make the healthiest choices possible. I'm going to break it down for you so your new diet of plant foods is totally doable and won't even disrupt your life too much.

I use the terms "plant-based" and "vegan" throughout this chapter. "Vegan" refers to food that is free of animal products. "Plant-based" refers to a vegan food that is whole and minimally processed. When it comes to a healthy heart, your diet should be as "plant-based" as possible, in that your meals should predominantly consist of whole, unprocessed foods, with only a small amount, if any, of minimally processed foods.

Assess What You Already Eat That Is Vegan

First, it's time to take a look at the vegan foods you are already eating. Chances are you already eat a decent amount of vegan food—and no, I don't mean just French fries! From fresh summer salads, to gorgeous pasta dishes with fresh marinara, to your mom's famous guacamole...these dishes are all vegan foods. When you reach for a snack of carrot and celery with hummus dip, you're eating vegan. The same goes for a peanut butter and jelly sandwich, which, admittedly, isn't the healthiest of options. But as you can see, delicious vegan food is likely already on your radar. We're just going to move these dishes a little closer to center stage. And there are so many substantial sources of plant-based protein that you're not going to feel that giving up animal products is a sacrifice on fullness or flavor!

Face the "Dreaded" Pantry Purge Head-on

Before you can fill your kitchen with new and wholesome plant-based foods, you've got to make some room—literally. This means doing a kitchen-wide purge of all non-vegan foods. It's best to complete this step in one fell swoop—that way you won't be tempted by lingering tubs of ice cream or hot dogs. Take an afternoon to pull out meat and dairy products to give away or otherwise remove from your fridge, pantry, and cabinets. If you are living with family members, roommates, or a partner who will continue eating these foods, at least dedicate some shelf and fridge space for your new sustenance. Don't worry about running short on great food options; in the next chapter, we will focus on the staples that will keep your cabinets full and your stomach happy.

Don't Focus on What You *Can't* Eat—Focus on What You *Can* Eat Instead

You'll go crazy if you fixate on the old foods that are no longer in your fridge and cabinets. So, once you get rid of your former foods, make a concerted effort not to spend too much thought on them; focusing on what you can't eat won't serve you in the long run.

Still, it's not unusual to get hit with a craving for meat or dairy. When this happens, ask yourself which plant-based meal might satisfy your craving. Your new diet allows for all kinds of delicious meals for you to enjoy and new foods to try. So when the urge for one of your former foods presents itself, whip up a crave-worthy plant-based dinner instead. You'll be delighted when you find plant foods that really do satisfy you, and eventually you will leave those old cravings in the past and start longing for your new healthier foods instead.

Become a Smart Ingredient Swapper

Adopting a plant-based diet involves a shift in the specific foods you prepare, but you can still eat in a way that is familiar to you. During your transition to a plant-based diet, it's helpful to assess the food you normally eat and figure out how to convert it to a plant-based meal instead. The good news: Sandwiches, soups, pastas, and more can remain on the menu. You'll simply swap out some ingredients for healthier plant-based substitutions. And though none of these foods require a meat or dairy substitute, sometimes while transitioning to a plant-based diet, it can be helpful to incorporate a vegan imitation meat or cheese as you're getting used to your new diet.

- **Stir-fry.** Easy enough! Instead of frying up meat, use tofu or seitan (a product with a meaty texture made from the protein of wheat) with vegetables and your favorite sauce.

- **Loaded baked potato.** Bring on the spuds. But this time, swap out cheese, bacon, and sour cream for salsa, avocado chunks, beans, or your favorite roasted vegetables.

- **A burger with "the works."** You can still bite into a tasty burger anytime you please. Try a black bean or veggie patty piled high with sautéed onions and roasted bell peppers. You can even top it with a slice of vegan cheese, if you require a tasty "melty" topping. Add a dollop of Dijon and you're all set.

- **Steak frites.** Trade in your usual steak for an oven-roasted marinated portobello mushroom with a balsamic reduction

123

glaze. Try sweet potato wedges dusted with chili powder, cumin, and sea salt for a twist on regular fries.

- **Kitchen sink salad.** Is your fridge overflowing with left-overs? Try an "everything but the sink" salad full of the veggies and ingredients in your fridge. Think beyond carrots and celery—add in fun ingredients like sauerkraut and chickpeas for crunch and flavor. Cut-up chunks of sweet potato make a surprisingly delicious addition to a salad too. Drizzle on a creamy tahini dressing and you'll never look back.

- **Pizza.** Who says a decadent pizza has to be a cholesterol-laden chunk of bread? Take a store-bought crust (or make your own), add tomato sauce and your favorite vegetables, and throw it in the oven. By the way, traditional Italian pizzas often do not have cheese. However, if you do crave something cheesy on top, there are delicious vegan cheeses that melt nicely.

- **Pasta.** Make a hearty bowl of pasta with a whole-wheat pasta, marinara sauce, roasted vegetables, and your favorite variety of beans. If you're accustomed to a "meaty" pasta sauce, consider adding something such as Gardein Ground Crumble or MorningStar Farms Grillers Crumbles.

Take Your Transition One Day at a Time and Move at Your Own Pace

As I've emphasized before, don't get overwhelmed by the magnitude of these changes you're making for your heart and your overall health. Slow and steady wins the race. Focus on what you can do today before you worry about long-term changes; the daily choices you make are what make up these changes in the first place. As long as you keep your focus solely on your next plant-based meal, you will be fine.

Everyone is different, so if you feel like you must make a gradual transition from your current diet to a plant-based diet, do whatever makes you feel comfortable. Maybe it's more practical for you to eat plant-based foods during the week and have small portions of meat and dairy on the weekends for a couple of months, until you fully adjust to your new diet. Just keep in mind that, eventually, you are aiming to eat only plant-based meals.

Allow for Setbacks on Your Food Journey

You're going to make some mistakes from time to time, and that's okay. Making any drastic dietary changes is a process, and it's unreasonable to expect perfection when you're starting out. Recommit each time you experience a slip-up. But be sure to keep some easy-to-prepare ingredients on hand for times when you are tempted to veer off course. (Think frozen vegan burritos, salad mix, frozen vegetables, and sauce to whip up into a quick stir-fry.)

Be a Gracious Guest

Your friends and family may not be aware that you've changed your diet. So whenever you have a dinner to attend, it's always a good idea to let your host know about your new way of eating. While some hosts will go out of their way to have plant-based options for you, many will not. If you're attending a potluck, ask your host what you can bring. I like to prepare a large salad with nuts, dried fruit, beans, lentils, or tofu for protein, and a unique dressing. This salad can serve as a side dish for the guests who may be eating meat as their main course, but can also serve as a satisfying meal for me.

Make a Game Plan for Dining Out

Dining at a vegetarian or vegan restaurant can be a great opportunity to try new foods without worrying about what on the menu might or might not contain animal products. Ethnic restaurants tend to have more plant-based options because their cultures often revolve less around meat as the center of the meal.

Most restaurants will have at least one vegan item on the menu. If not, there is typically something that can be "vegan-ized." For instance, you could order a vegetable pizza without cheese, or a garden salad with garbanzo beans added. Even a steakhouse can prepare a good vegan meal. At a recent professional meeting at a local steakhouse, I received a huge plate of some of the most delicious roasted vegetables that my omnivorous friends ogled with envy!

While you can always ask your server what is or is not vegan, often I like to call ahead. It can be uncomfortable to try and tease out exactly what is or is not vegan on a menu during a date or when dining with people you don't know well. Also, I hate to put a server on the spot, since she may not know whether an item is vegan. It's easier to sort it out over the phone before arriving at the restaurant.

Watch out for non-vegan ingredients that can sneak their way into food; often butter can be used for sautéing vegetables or brushed onto bread, or eggs may be added in various breads and crusts. A chicken or beef broth may be used to flavor a dish, and lard is sometimes used as a shortening, particularly in

Mexican restaurants. If you're suspicious, ask directly about the ingredient. For example, at a Mexican restaurant, you may ask if the refried beans are vegan, and the server might say, "Yes." I will often follow that up with, "What are the beans fried in? Is there any lard?" Sometimes the server will admit that, yes, the beans are fried in lard. It's always best to be specific when you ask, because it's easy to give a blanket "yes" answer when asked if a food is vegan.

However, errors occur, despite your best efforts. I can recall a recent dinner where I made it clear that I was vegan, and asked specifically if a dish was vegan, only to have it arrive with plenty of cheese on it. Certainly, this can be infuriating, and I try my best to be patient when I send the dish back. Do your best to be good natured about these slip-ups—most restaurants truly want to do their best to accommodate you.

Take a Culinary Journey Around the World

Ethnic restaurants often have great plant-based food selections. The next time you're making dinner plans, consider trying one of these vegan-friendly options:

• Thai

• Middle Eastern

• Indian

• Ethiopian

• Greek

• Chinese

There are also great online resources for vegan options at chain restaurants. For more information, refer to PETA's fast food recommendations: www.peta.org/living/food/chain-restaurants.

Keep Some Perspective and a Sense of Humor

While your diet and health is a serious matter, try not to take it so seriously that you lose your sense of joy surrounding the gift of food. Eating is a significant part of life. Food is necessary for survival, but it is also ceremonial; it's a reason to gather with loved ones and the foundation of milestones like weddings, anniversaries, and birthdays. So keep this in mind as you face the challenges of eating a plant-based diet—because at some point you will probably deal with funny looks from people, and you'll occasionally have to work a little harder to find appropriate food options than your friends who eat meat and dairy. If you can laugh your way through awkward moments, you will be much happier overall.

Also keep this in mind: Whenever someone is teasing you about your choices, often that comes from their own sense of curiosity, and even an insecurity about their own choices. So laugh along with them, and stay open to sharing your experiences with them, because one day they too may cross over to the vegan side. I've seen it happen plenty of times.

How to Gracefully Face Questions from Others

That brings me to my next topic: You will be asked at some point, *Why are you eating this way? What's wrong with a good burger?* There's no reason for you to have to preach about the destruction of the environment, the scourge of diseases related to a meat- and dairy-heavy diet, or the torture of animals. In a casual setting, I keep my answer short: *Animal foods lead to the diseases that I treat. Also, I care about animals and I want to be healthy.* If they want to know more than that, then they can ask. People will be turned off if they feel judged, so I try to frame it from the perspective of *This is why I chose this lifestyle*—not that people who eat meat are bad.

Next up we will cover the foods that belong in your new plant-based kitchen! This is where the real fun begins, because you now get to explore new ways to eat the tasty and exciting foods that can heal your heart and body.

CHAPTER 10

The Stress-Free Guide to a Well-Stocked Vegan Kitchen

By now, you should be ready to fill your pantry, freezer, and fridge with healthy and delicious plant-based foods. I believe in keeping plenty of fresh and non-perishable ingredients on hand so you can always whip up something healthy and delicious whenever hunger or culinary inspiration strikes. Below, I've broken down the essential components of a vegan kitchen. Feel free to use this chapter as a jumping-off point for your exploration into the world of plant-based food. Have fun, keep an open mind, and enjoy the culinary journey to better health.

Veggies

Filled with vitamins, nutrients, and fiber, along with a multitude of phytochemicals and micronutrients, vegetables should fill half your lunch and dinner plate. And yet, they are often the most neglected category of food in the diet. Sadly, only 26 percent of the U.S. population gets three or more servings of vegetables daily, and countless others barely eat even one vegetable daily.[1]

I'm often asked if vegetables should be purchased fresh or frozen, and whether frozen vegetables are less healthy than fresh veggies. Either is fine. In fact, frozen vegetables may have more of their nutrients because they are harvested and then frozen at their peak freshness, sealing in nutrients. I buy plenty of vegetables weekly at the farmers market, but I like to have some frozen vegetables on hand to use in a pinch.

Given the health benefits of veggies, if you're not a veggie eater, it's time to become one. Start with the vegetables that you do like and eat more of them. Also, know that vegetables can be "disguised" in food. Add shredded carrots in a marinara sauce, or a handful of spinach in a fruit smoothie (you can't even taste it!). Or you can put a veggie burger on top of a bed of leafy greens instead of on a bun.

- Squash
- Zucchini
- Radishes
- Cabbage
- Eggplant
- Arugula
- Lettuce
- Carrots
- Kale
- Spinach

Fruits

I love fruit! It's a naturally sweet treat that's loaded with nutrients. And yet, only 32 percent of the U.S. population eats two servings of fruit daily.[2]

Like vegetables, fresh or frozen fruits are fine; it just depends on your preference. I like to pick up local, in-season fruit from my farmers market. I buy apples and pears in the winter, stone fruit like peaches and plums in the summer, and persimmons, my favorite fruit, which are abundant in Southern California, in the fall. I'll shop my local market for bananas, which are not indigenous to this area. And, because I'm not a big fan of cutting up fruit, I like to buy frozen mango and pineapple, which can easily be put it in a bowl and microwaved on a low setting for a few seconds to defrost, or frozen berries, which are an easy addition to a hot oatmeal.

I tend to eat fruit earlier in the day, but whatever time of day works for you is fine. Often, I start my day with a fruit and vegetable smoothie, which is a great way to easily drink a few servings of fruit and even a couple servings of vegetables. Also, I like to keep a piece of fruit, like an apple or persimmon, on hand for a quick snack during the day. As always, sample lots of different fruits and see which work for you.

- Mango
- Pineapple
- Peaches
- Plums
- Persimmons
- Apples
- Pears
- Strawberries
- Bananas

Some Perspective on Organics

Organic foods are grown without pesticides, synthetic fertilizer, genetically modified organisms, sewage sludge, or ionizing radiation. It is thought by many that organic foods are healthier and may contain more nutrients. Also, organic methods of growing food are better for the health of the soil.

Some produce tends to have higher amounts of pesticide residue, and these fruits and vegetables may, in fact, be better to purchase organic. To learn more, see the Environmental Working Group's "Dirty Dozen" list at www.ewg.org/foodnews/dirty_dozen_list.php.[3] I would also recommend that you buy organic soy milk or tofu, as the majority of soybeans grown in the U.S. are genetically modified. Genetically modified food has been present only since 1994, and there is a lot that we do not know about its effects on our health.

However, don't let a focus on organic food keep you from eating healthfully. If you can afford to purchase organics, then include organic produce in your shopping cart. Organic is a great option. But it's more important to make sure you're actually getting your fruits and veggies.

Nuts and Seeds

Nuts and seeds contain protein, fiber, B vitamins, vitamin E, and many are great sources of omega-3 fatty acids. They also contain monounsaturated fats. You can eat them straight up, or in the form of a delicious nut butter, like peanut butter or almond butter.

A small handful of nuts can be a great snack. I find a banana with almond butter quite filling before a morning workout. I also like to add a sprinkle of chia seeds or flax seeds to my oatmeal for an omega-3 boost.

While nuts and seeds are full of nutrients, they are also packed with calories, so take care not to "go nuts" and eat too many servings at once. A small handful may have about 200 calories, and it can be easy to eat several times that amount in one sitting. I like to purchase Trader Joe's individual packets of nuts, which each have 200 calories.

Also, when purchasing nut butters, choose items whose only ingredients are nuts, salt, and water. Many popular brands of nut butter, particularly peanut butter, have added sugars and oil, making them less healthy choices.

- Cashews
- Pecans
- Walnuts
- Almonds
- Peanuts
- Macadamia nuts
- Pistachios
- Sunflower seeds
- Chia seeds
- Flax seeds

The diet of Dr. Caldwell Esselstyn's studies of patients with coronary artery disease excluded nuts, seeds, oil, and avocados from the diet. This has been demonstrated to be an effective diet at preventing and reversing heart disease, and is reasonable. I do not instruct my patients to shun these foods, but rather to watch their portion sizes; after all, nuts and seeds do contain vitamins and minerals and healthy fats. Further, if you have not been diagnosed with arterial disease, there is no reason why you need to subscribe to an oil-free and nut-free diet.

Legumes and Pulses

Lentils and beans have plenty of soluble fiber, protein, carbohydrates, folate, and iron. They pack plenty of flavor and can be added to soups, stews, salads, or turned into a delicious homemade hummus.

Beans can be purchased dry or canned. If you have the time to soak and cook your beans, this may be the tastiest option. Sometimes I will do this, but I also like to have a couple of cans on hand. Trader Joe's has steamed lentils in a bag that are ready to eat, and I like to mix these with their store brand bruschetta or add them to a salad—yum!

Some people avoid beans because of fear of flatulence, which is understandable. However, know that as your body gets used to these, your gaseous issues will gradually resolve.

- Pinto beans
- Garbanzo beans
- Kidney beans
- Lentils
- Black beans
- Adzuki beans

Grains

Whole grains are a great source of B vitamins and fiber, which is important for keeping your bowels healthy. The fiber in whole grains may also help to lower cholesterol and blood pressure and help you to feel full.

Oatmeal is one of my favorite foods, and can be prepared quickly as instant oats, or for a richer texture can be cooked longer, like steel cut oats. While quinoa is a "pseudo grain" since it is technically a seed, it cooks quickly, has plenty of protein, and is a great choice on a salad or to add to a stir-fry.

- Rice
- Oats
- Barley
- Quinoa
- Whole wheat
- Polenta
- Couscous
- Amaranth

Plant Proteins

As a vegan, I'm often asked, "Where do you get your protein?" Trust me, it's easy enough. While beans, whole grains, nuts, seeds, and even vegetables have protein, tofu, seitan, and tempeh are the most concentrated in protein.

Tofu is versatile and can be purchased in a soft form to make soups or sauces, or in firmer varieties, which work better in stir-fries. Baked flavored tofu can be cut up in squares and added to salads. I recommend buying organic tofu (see organic sidebar).

Seitan is made from wheat gluten, which is the protein portion of wheat. It has a "meaty" texture and goes well in stews or stir-fries. Tempeh is made from fermented soybeans, is quite versatile, and I've even seen it used as a "fake bacon" on sandwiches.

- Tofu
- Seitan
- Tempeh

Herbs and Spices

Herbs (either fresh or dried) and spices are an amazing way to "spice up" your dishes and bring vibrant flavor to your cooking. They bring warmth, coolness, bitterness, pungency, or earthiness to foods and can be truly transformative—not to mention, they're good for you! Be sure to experiment with these flavor-enhancing wonders to take your meals to new heights.

- Basil
- Garlic
- Pepper
- Thyme
- Sage
- Oregano
- Rosemary
- Cilantro
- Chives
- Allspice
- Cardamom
- Turmeric
- Cinnamon
- Ginger
- Cumin

Oils

In vegan cooking, you will still probably have occasion to cook with and consume plant-based oils, so it's important to know which ones are best. Some oils are considered to be healthier choices, such as olive, canola, avocado, or grapeseed oils, because they contain more monounsaturated fats (the "good for you" kind of fats). Oils are a better choice for cooking than solid fats, such as butter, shortening, or lard. However, oil is pure fat, and is very dense in calories, so if you choose to use oil in your cooking, use it sparingly. Vegetable stock (see sidebar) or even water can serve as an alternative if you prefer cooking without oil, but you will need to adjust your recipe accordingly so you still produce a tasty meal.

- Extra virgin olive oil
- Canola oil
- Avocado oil
- Grapeseed oil

Vegan Condiments

I like to have some basic condiments on hand. It's easy to add these to a recipe for flavor. If you're more ambitious, you can make your own salad dressings, and there are plenty of great recipes on the internet to inspire you. My favorite is a miso dressing from the farmers market. I also love adding soy sauce and rice vinegar to a stir-fry.

- Soy sauce
- Salad dressings
- Pasta sauce
- Marinades
- Rice vinegar
- Cider vinegar

Vegetable Stock: A Healthy Kitchen Staple

I love to keep homemade vegetable stock on hand because it's versatile and delicious! I will typically prepare it on a day when I'm doing a lot of cooking. I take my vegetable scraps, such as beet greens, the ends of zucchini, leftover onions, and whatever else I have on hand and throw it in a pot with a strainer along with water and salt. I'll cover the pot and let it simmer for a little over an hour. At the end of that time, I'll have a delicious vegetable broth!

I like to use the broth for soups, such as a vegan matza ball soup that I prepare every year for Passover. Or, I will use it for making stews, adding cornstarch to thicken it up, or for flavoring a stir-fry. You can even add a few tablespoons of veggie stock in the place of oil when you need a healthy liquid for pan cooking vegetables. It stores well in the fridge for about a week, or you can freeze broth cubes in an ice tray to make small portions for recipes.

My Favorite Brands of Pre-packaged Food

For those moments when you need to grab a pre-prepared bite, these are my favorite brands of vegan convenience foods. Let me stress that these items—however tasty—are still *processed* foods, and while they are vegan, they are quite high in sodium. These should be considered occasional treats; they are not ideal foods for everyday consumption. If you are someone who is watching your sodium consumption due to any health issues, you should be very cautious when consuming anything on this list. Instead, you should stick primarily to healthy, fresh meals prepared at home from scratch. That way, you can control the sodium levels and the other ingredients.

- Gardein *Mandarin Orange Crispy Chick'n*
- Beyond Meat *The Beyond Burger*—This is my favorite veggie burger. It has a very meaty texture.
- Trader Joe's *Meatless Meatballs*
- Trader Joe's *Roasted Vegetable Pizza*
- Tofurky *Deli Slices*—These come in a variety of flavors and are great for sandwiches and wraps.
- Amy's—The entire Amy's line of food is vegetarian, with many vegan options. They have great pot pies, burritos, and other quick meals.

Helpful Kitchen Tips

Be a prepping pro. Spend a few minutes chopping and washing your vegetables after you buy them. This makes planning meals a piece of cake.

Busy week ahead? Do some batch cooking. Batch cooking involves cooking many meals all at once, and it can greatly reduce your cooking responsibilities during the week. I like to batch cook on a Tuesday night when I get home from the farmers market and my veggies are fresh.

Get the kids involved. Even if other family members continue to eat meat and dairy, you can still be a shining example of good health. Ask your children to help you with easy food prep responsibilities like washing and trimming veggies or choosing new recipes for the week. It's never too early to start setting an example for good nutrition.

Make the most of farmers markets. I love my local farmers market! I'm a regular at the Sherman Oaks Farmers Market, which is held in the parking lot of a local mall every Tuesday evening. I stop off there after work and pick up most of the fruits and vegetables that I will eat for the week. One local vendor has the best heirloom tomatoes I've ever eaten. Another has Japanese sweet potatoes that I like to chop up and add to my salads. Another is a Korean vendor who sells all vegan products, including kimchi (which often is prepared in fish brine and therefore off limits), daikon radish, burdock, ucha greens, and all sorts of good stuff you may have never heard of. They also make a delicious oil-free miso dressing and a brown rice-based protein called tempha that I like to add to my salads. The produce is local and fresh, and in my opinion is tastier than what I can get in a grocery store. Make the effort to find a nearby farmers market and check them out. You won't be disappointed!

Essential Tools and Appliances

A few good, sharp knives. Only recently have I discovered how much easier it is to cook when you have good, sharp knives and know how to use them. A quality knife set doesn't need to be expensive. With good knives and proper technique, your food prep will be far more efficient.

High-speed blender or food processor. I love my Vitamix!!!! It's a high-speed blender that can pulverize anything. It makes great smoothies, can "rice" cauliflower, make soups, or even a banana-based frozen dessert treat. High-speed blenders are well worth the investment, and allow you to make easy work of blending tough vegetables, frozen fruits, and anything in between.

A food processor is equally useful in chopping your produce for easy meal prep.

Steamer baskets. Bamboo steamers are excellent for cooking food quickly. Just drop in your veggies, cover with the lid, and place the basket over a pan of simmering water. In about ten minutes, you'll have delicious steamed vegetables ready to eat. I like to cook red peppers, cabbage, and baby carrots using this method.

Salad spinner. A salad spinner is a super useful and inexpensive kitchen tool that makes washing leafy veggies a snap. It quickly cleans lettuce, herbs, kale, and even fruit. You can even use it to store your salad greens until you need them. Just rinse them, spin them dry, and store them in the fridge inside the spinner.

Compost pail. You are about to start producing a lot of scraps, so you may want to compost them to enrich your garden or lawn. I keep an air-tight bin on my kitchen counter for scraps and empty it into my composter in the backyard every few days. I use the compost for my fruit trees and my backyard garden. At any rate, a compost pail with a sturdy lid will help you manage veggie remnants like potato peels, onion skins, and celery hearts.

By now I hope you are eager to join the ranks of plant-eating enthusiasts everywhere! Now that you are armed with all this new information on how to eat your way to a healthier heart and body, your life is about to change in remarkable ways. Your kitchen will be the site of many upcoming adventures as you prepare a delicious assortment of heart healthy meals. To get you started, I've included some of my favorite recipes for exceptionally great plant-based dishes. It is my hope that these recipes fuel inspiration, excitement, and gratitude for the many exciting and nutritious meals in your future.

Grab a fork, because here we go!

CHAPTER 11

Recipes

Disclaimer: As you read earlier in this book, Dr. Caldwell Esselstyn's work demonstrated the benefits of a strictly whole-food plant-based diet that was free of oil, avocados, nuts, and seeds. In the population studied, which consisted of patients with disease of their coronary arteries, this diet demonstrated dramatic reversal of plaque in the arteries and improvement in parameters of health such as blood pressure, cholesterol levels, and body weight.

The recipes in this section may contain oil, nuts, or seeds. If you choose to follow Esselstyn's diet, you can eliminate these ingredients, or I provide oil-free alternatives for the recipes.

Finally, I am not a chef. I'm a busy full-time cardiologist who likes to prepare healthy meals quickly in my kitchen. These are not elaborate recipes, nor are they necessarily gourmet dinners. They're quick and easy. There are plenty of resources online and a myriad of vegan cookbooks, so if you want to take your cooking to the next level, that would be your next step.

Morning Recipes

TOFU SCRAMBLE

A tofu scramble is a great way to start your day with plenty of energy. This breakfast is packed with protein from the tofu and plenty of antioxidants and nutrients from the vegetables. If you want to make this dish without oil, you can sauté the onion in a bit of water.

Ingredients: | **Serves two.**

14 oz. firm or extra-firm tofu, drained and mashed with a fork into crumbly pieces

1 medium sweet potato, chopped into small cubes

2 cups fresh spinach, or 1 cup frozen

1 medium red pepper, diced

1 medium onion, chopped

1-2 cloves garlic, minced

1-2 tbsp. Bragg liquid amino acids or soy sauce

1 tbsp. olive oil

1 tsp. turmeric

1/2 tsp. paprika

pepper to taste

Directions: Heat oil in a skillet. Add the onion and sauté until translucent. Add garlic, sweet potato, spinach, and red pepper. Add Bragg or soy sauce, turmeric, and paprika. Add mashed tofu. Sauté, stirring occasionally, for 10-12 minutes. Serve warm.

TROPICAL BREAKFAST QUINOA

Oatmeal isn't the only whole grain that can be cooked up in a bowl for breakfast! If I have leftover quinoa from dinner, I'll easily mix it with some frozen fruit and a nut milk and enjoy it for breakfast.

Ingredients: | **Serves two.**

1/2 cup dry quinoa

1/2 cup coconut milk

1 cup mango, chopped

1 cup pineapple, chopped

1 tbsp. chia seeds

Directions: First, cook the quinoa. Bring 1 cup of water to a boil, and add quinoa. Then turn the heat down to low and simmer for 15 minutes. Next, turn off the heat and allow the quinoa to rest for 5 minutes. Then, fluff the quinoa with a fork and transfer to a large bowl. Add soy milk, mango, pineapple, and chia seeds and mix. This dish can be served hot or cold.

GREEN SMOOTHIE

A smoothie is a great way to start your day with some fruits and vegetables. This is my standard recipe. If you don't yet eat a lot of vegetables, or you're new to green smoothies, you may want to add less vegetables and more fruit until your palate adapts. Carrots and bananas add sweetness to this recipe. Often, I'll mix up the fruits and vegetables based on what I have on hand. Zucchini, beets, or even a little bit of lettuce (not a lot because it's bitter) can blend into a smoothie quite well.

Ingredients: | **Serves one.**

3/4 cup unsweetened plant milk (I like coconut milk or almond milk)

1 cup kale

3 oz. carrots

1 banana

1 stalk celery

5 ice cubes

Directions: Place ingredients in a high-power blender and blend until smooth.

GREEN ALMOND SMOOTHIE

This very filling smoothie has almond butter for healthy fats, chia seeds for omega-3, and maca powder for plenty of energy. It is great for breakfast or for a pre- or post-workout snack.

Ingredients: | **Serves one.**

1 cup spinach

1 cup unsweetened coconut milk

1 banana

1 tbsp. almond butter

1/2 tbsp. chia seeds

1/2 tbsp. maca powder

2 medjool dates

Directions: Blend all ingredients in a Vitamix or other blender and drink up.

"Anytime" Meals

BUTTERNUT SQUASH SOUP

This simple but filling soup is a great warm meal for a cold day.

Ingredients: | **Serves two.**

1/2 medium-sized butternut squash, cut length-wise, seeds removed

2 tsp. miso

3/4 cup water

Directions: Preheat your oven to 350 degrees. Place butternut squash, cut side down, in a glass tray, filled with one inch of water. Bake for about 45 minutes, or until squash is soft. Allow squash to cool. Once cooled, scoop squash into Vitamix, high-powered blender, or food processor. Add miso and water. On the Vitamix, if there is a "soup" setting, just start the mixer in that setting and by the end you will have hot soup. On any other device, puree until well mixed and warm.

RICED CAULIFLOWER

"Riced" cauliflower can take the place of rice on your dinner plate and is an easy way to sneak a vegetable into your repertoire. This dish goes great with stir-fry or chili—or it can be eaten on its own.

Ingredients: | **Serves four as a side dish.**

1 small head of cauliflower

1 tbsp. olive oil

1/4 tsp. Himalayan sea salt

pepper, to taste

Directions: "Rice" the cauliflower by breaking into small pieces and blending in a Vitamix or other blender at low setting. Add only a handful of cauliflower at a time to the blender. Cauliflower should be blended until it takes on the consistency of rice. Next, heat oil at medium heat in a skillet. Add riced cauliflower, salt, and pepper to skillet. Sauté for about 8 minutes. Serve hot.

CHILI

A warm bowl of chili on a cold day serves as a perfect meal. This recipe, with sweet potatoes, bulgur, veggies, and beans will fill you up and keep you full.

Ingredients: | **Serves six.**

2 cups veggie broth

1 28 oz. can Muir Glen fire roasted diced tomatoes

1 15 oz. can black beans, rinsed

1 15 oz. can kidney beans, rinsed

2 medium sweet potatoes, without skin, diced

1/2 cup frozen sweet corn

1 red bell pepper, diced

1 medium zucchini, diced

1/2 cup uncooked bulgur

2 tsp. pepper

1 tbsp. cumin

1 tbsp. curry powder

1 small onion

1 tbsp. hot sauce

Salt to taste

Directions: Add all ingredients to a crock pot and cook on high for two hours. Once done cooking, blend ingredients on low setting in a Vitamix until it reaches a chili-like consistency.

LASAGNA

I love preparing this hearty dish for a big family dinner. You can vary the vegetables in the recipe; I've also used zucchini or sweet potato for a different flavor.

Ingredients: | Serves six.

12 dry lasagna noodles (not cooked)

1 jar marinara sauce (I like Trader Joe's organic tomato basil marinara)

2 cups carrots, shredded

1 14 oz. package of firm or extra-firm tofu

Juice of 1/2 lemon

2 cups of chopped broccoli, spinach, or any other green vegetable

Daiya mozzarella cheese (optional)

Directions: Preheat oven to 350 degrees. In a glass lasagna tray, spoon some of the marinara sauce to cover the bottom. Then place three lasagna noodles over the sauce. Layer the shredded carrots on next.

Drain the liquid from the tofu and then place the tofu in a Vitamix or blender. Add lemon juice, and blend on low setting until tofu takes on the consistency of ricotta cheese. Layer the tofu mixture on top of the carrots.

Place three more lasagna noodles on top of the tofu mixture. Add broccoli or spinach. Pour sauce on top.

Layer on three more lasagna noodles. Pour the remainder of the marinara sauce on top. Then sprinkle on the optional Daiya cheese.

Cover the lasagna in foil and place it in the oven. After 25 minutes, remove the foil. Cook for a total of 50 minutes, or until noodles are soft and the center of the lasagna is warm.

PARTY SALAD

This is my go-to recipe to bring to a potluck. Most of the salad will be ingredients from my local farmers market, though I do add a couple of prepared items for flavor. Flavorful as a side dish, but can be filling enough as an entrée if there are no good plant-based options. The key to any party salad is to make it unique—I like to add fresh fruit, dried fruit, candied nuts, and cubed baked Japanese sweet potatoes, and serve with a vinaigrette on the side.

Ingredients: | **Serves six.**

3 cups lettuce

2 large heirloom tomatoes, chopped

4 small Persian cucumbers, diced

3 carrots, shredded

2 tablespoons ground flax seeds

1 large Japanese sweet potato, baked, peeled, and diced into small cubes of about 1/2 inch

1 apple or pear, sliced

1/2 cup dried cranberries

1/2 cup Trader Joe's cinnamon roasted almonds

Directions: Mix ingredients in a bowl. Serve with a raspberry vinaigrette on the side. The salad is sweet and flavorful enough on its own that you may not even want to add dressing.

PASTA PRIMAVERA

This tasty pasta is another great option for a potluck. I don't always use the same vegetables each time I prepare this dish; often I'll just take whatever is on hand in my refrigerator. For protein, you can add beans or store-bought imitation meatballs (Trader Joe's makes a great vegan meatball).

Ingredients: | **Serves four as a main dish.**

1 box pasta, cooked

1 jar of marinara sauce

1/4 cup vegetable broth or 2 tbsp. olive oil

1 medium onion, diced

2 cloves garlic, minced

1 cup mushrooms, sliced

1 medium zucchini, sliced

1 yellow pepper, sliced

Directions: In a large saucepan, heat the vegetable broth or olive oil at medium heat. Once the pan is hot, add the onion and sautée until translucent. Add the garlic and sautée for about 3 minutes. Next, add mushrooms, zucchini, and yellow pepper. Sprinkle with salt and pepper to taste. Once vegetables are cooked, add sauce and cook for a couple minutes. Add this sauce mixture to your cooked pasta and serve hot.

TOFU STIR-FRY

This stir-fry recipe is pretty versatile. The vegetables I chose this time were the ones I had on hand; it just so happens that my backyard garden had a couple of green peppers ready to go! But, eggplant also goes well in this—it just requires a bit longer cooking. Sliced mushrooms are also a great choice for a stir-fry. To make this oil-free, use either water or a little bit of Bragg's or soy sauce when heating the wok or skillet.

Ingredients: | **Serves four.**

1 14 oz. package of firm or extra-firm tofu, drained and cut into cubes

2 cups spinach, rinsed

1 green pepper, chopped

1 red pepper, chopped

2 cups broccoli florets, cut to pieces no more than one inch in diameter

1 medium onion, coarsely chopped

2 cloves garlic, minced

1 tbsp. olive oil

2 tbsp. Bragg's or soy sauce

1 tbsp. rice vinegar

Directions: In a wok or large skillet, heat oil. Add onion and sautée until translucent. Turn the heat to medium-low. Add garlic and sautée until it starts to darken. Add Bragg's and rice vinegar. Next add broccoli and peppers. Add spinach. Once the spinach is wilted, add tofu. Stir frequently, and cook for an additional 7-10 minutes. Serve with rice, cauliflower rice, pasta, quinoa, or your favorite grain.

YELLOW CURRY

I love Thai food. This tasty curry recipe is a great way to bring it home.

Ingredients: | **Serves four.**

1 14 oz. package of extra-firm tofu, cut into 1/2-inch cubes

1 tbsp. oil (can use water to stir-fry instead)

1 can of full-fat coconut milk

2 moderate-sized sweet potatoes, peeled and chopped into 1/2-inch cubes

1 head of broccoli, chopped into florets

1/2 pound of mushrooms

1 onion, peeled and coarsely chopped

2 tbsp. Bragg liquid aminos

1 tbsp. Thai Kitchen red curry paste

2 tsp. curry powder

1 tsp. salt

1/2 tsp. cumin (optional)

1 tsp. turmeric

1/4 cup cornstarch to thicken

1 tbsp. Sriracha, or to taste

Directions: Heat oil (or water) in a large skillet. Add onions and cook until translucent. Add 2 cups water, bring to a boil, and add the sweet potatoes. Cook for 10 minutes. Add mushrooms, broccoli, and tofu, and cook for 5 minutes.

Then add coconut milk, Bragg liquid aminos, red curry paste, salt, Sriracha, and spices. Cook together for 5 minutes. Finally, add cornstarch to thicken. Serve over brown rice.

Quick Snacks

CANNELLINI BEAN HUMMUS

Cannellini beans are my favorite choice for making hummus. I like to serve this for impromptu gatherings since it's so easy to throw together. It's a great crowd-pleaser.

Ingredients: | Serves six.

1 can cannellini beans, drained and rinsed

2 tbsp. oil (can be omitted)

2 tbsp. tahini

1/4 tsp. salt

1/4 tsp. ground cumin

2 medium-sized garlic cloves, chopped

1/4 cup water (less or more depending on your desired consistency)

Directions: Blend ingredients in a Vitamix on medium setting until hummus reaches a smooth consistency. Pour in a serving bowl and garnish with sprinkled cumin and pine nuts. Serve with cut up veggies or pita chips.

TEXAS CAVIAR

This Texas caviar is one of my favorite party recipes and is great for a mid-afternoon snack. Date syrup is a natural alternative to white sugar and can be found at health food stores or at ethnic grocery stores such as Middle Eastern, Jewish, or Armenian grocers. Texas caviar is delicious on its own or great with chips or dipped vegetables.

Ingredients: | **Serves six.**

1 red pepper, diced into small pieces

1 green pepper, diced

1 cup sweet frozen corn, thawed, or 1 can corn, rinsed

1/4 cup green onion, diced

1/4 cup cilantro, diced

1/2 cup white vinegar

3 tbsp. date syrup

1 jalapeño, diced (optional)

Directions: Mix all ingredients in a large bowl. Allow to chill in refrigerator for several hours or overnight before serving.

THE VEGAN HEART DOCTOR'S GUIDE

CHOCOLATE BANANA "ICE CREAM"

Here's a decadent replacement for standard ice cream that's healthy for you!

Ingredients: | **Serves two.**

2 bananas, sliced into bite-sized pieces and frozen

1/2 cup unsweetened coconut milk

1/2 tsp. cocoa

Directions: Add bananas, coconut, and cocoa to Vitamix. Process these ingredients using the "frozen desserts" Vitamix setting or a medium to high setting on a high-powered blender. Use the tamper to press down frozen bananas into the blade. Mix until ingredients are combined smoothly, or if in the "frozen desserts" mode, when the machine stops.

The "ice cream" can be eaten immediately, or for a harder consistency like packed ice cream, you can put the ingredients in a glass container, cover, freeze for an hour, scoop, and serve.

SECTION IV

Whole-Hearted Living

The Art of Whole-Hearted Living

In this book, we have covered the foundational aspects that can bring you and your heart back to a state of good health. You have learned what it means to take heart disease seriously, and now you have the tools to address it through healthcare, exercise, and diet. Finally, it's time to put the last puzzle piece into place by committing to achieve balance and peace in your body, mind, and soul.

There's a well-accepted connection between excess stress, anxiety, depression, and heart disease. While there needs to be more study on the subject, it's fairly clear that unmanaged stress creates physiological changes that can contribute to heart disease. What's more, the unhealthy way people attempt to handle this stress—smoking, overeating, avoiding exercise, etc.—exacerbates the problem.

Maintaining a healthy life balance is the solution to handling stress and dealing with harmful emotions. I see the truth of this in observing my patients and also my own life. This healthy balance is what allows me to thrive in my busy yet satisfying lifestyle. The same is true for all of us. Without balance, we cannot be our best selves each day.

For instance, if my life were only about the challenging work I do, then I would miss out on the other joys that bring me fulfillment. And while I do feel a tremendous sense of purpose from helping to heal my patients, I realize that I also need other factors to be truly happy—among them reflection, the pursuit of good health, rest, and time for fun with friends and loved ones.

The final chapter ahead is about making room in your life for your health, your work, and your happiness. When you can master the art of living each day with purpose, gratitude, and zest, your life will take on new dimensions—and your good health will allow you to appreciate and enjoy it all the more. Join me now on the journey to whole-hearted living.

CHAPTER 12

Going "Whole-Heart": Making the Journey to Total Wellness, Balance, and Peace

Upon reading this book, you have learned the "mechanical" basics that will help you return to excellent heart health and happiness and regain your vitality. Now we are going to talk about some other aspects of your life that impact your mental and emotional well-being, which of course connects back to your physical health. (It all works together!)

First, let's explore the concept of optimal health as it relates to your overall wellness. Physical health is really a spectrum, and while many of us can't expect to achieve totally "perfect" health, we can all certainly benefit from moving toward the healthy end of the continuum. But when you are facing heart disease or any other illness, this effort can feel like a scary uphill struggle. It can seem like physical wellness is far out of your reach, as well as the happiness and excitement that we all long to experience on the journey. Frankly, this is a false belief born out of fear, and I want you to refuse to believe it.

I see too many patients get discouraged about their health and give up on *everything*. They let their lack of physical health limit their entire lives—and as a result, they lose their joy, their spark, and their hope. Know this: If you follow the advice in this book, your health will improve. But keep in mind that even if achieving so-called "perfect health" were possible, you would still be on a journey full of challenges, ups and downs, and uncertainties. My wish is that you work hard to improve your physical health while you also seek happiness, meaning, peace, and purpose…because there is more than one way to repair a damaged heart.

I am referring to the *other* approach to wellness—the kind of healing that doesn't happen in the doctor's office or by exercising and improving your diet. I call this process going "whole-heart." It's about achieving wellness by putting every aspect of your life into perspective and balance, all for the good of your body, mind, and soul. Going whole-heart is a lifelong process that you should continue pursuing even after you get your heart disease markers in check, lower your weight and blood pressure, embrace better fitness, and adopt a healthier diet. It is meant to work in tandem with the health and nutritional guidelines already laid out in this book.

The guidelines in this chapter can give you the whole-hearted picture of wellness that will supercharge your energy and further fuel your journey toward physical wellness. While every healing aspect I cover may not resonate with you personally, I urge you to incorporate what works best and leave the rest.

Adopt these routines into your life to help you reach your highest wellness potential.

Spend time in nature. As I've mentioned before, it's very important to spend regular time outside. This practice combats our unnatural tendency to live artificial indoor lives, and it also just feels great to take in fresh air and sunshine on a regular basis.

Wherever you may live, find the most natural areas nearby and explore them regularly. This may include going on hikes or trail walks (and trail jogs!), kayaking, swimming, and more. Even here in busy Los Angeles we have Griffith Park, the country's largest park contained within a city, the Santa Monica Mountains, and even the beaches by the ocean.

Commit to adequate sleep and rest. The amount of sleep a person needs varies from individual to individual. I personally function best when I have about 7-8 hours of sleep, but others may need smaller or greater amounts to feel rested and refreshed. However much you need, make sleep a priority. I'm careful to never sacrifice sleep for workouts, even in the midst of training for important races. And if I have a poor night's sleep, or get called to the cath lab for an emergency angioplasty at 2:00 a.m., I certainly won't be making it to a 6:00 a.m. swim workout.

Of course, it's not always easy to get good, quality sleep when life gets in the way of your rest. Here are some tips to help you get the rest you need.

- **First, develop a healthy sleep routine.** If you want to consistently get a good night's sleep, start working now to form healthy bedtime habits. Go to bed around the same time and wake up about the same time every day. Make an effort to wind down in the hour or two before bedtime. And stay away from caffeine in the afternoon as that can disrupt your sleep.

- **Invest in some blackout curtains.** Blackout curtains block out most, or all, of the light from the street, the moon, or the neighbor's porch light. You'll be amazed at the difference a pitch-black room makes for your sleep.

- **Turn down the thermostat.** A cool room helps you drift off to sleep, so dial down the temperature at night in accordance with your comfort level.

- **Keep the television and computer out of your room.** Get rid of distractions like TV and the internet in your bedroom. If you devote this space mainly to sleeping, you'll be less likely to end up wide awake at bedtime.

- **Diffuse a relaxing essential oil.** Many people enjoy the scents of essential oils for relaxation. Try diffusing lavender or bergamot essential oil for a restful night.

- **Use a sound spa machine.** If ambient noise keeps you awake, consider using a sound spa to drown out the outside world. Many sound spas feature soundtracks of rain, ocean waves, or a steady hum to lull you to dreamland.

Build strong relationships. Our human need for connection is important and constant. Isolation and loneliness are both hard on the heart. You need loving relationships with other living beings, and there are plenty of ways to forge these connections. You can nurture caring relationships with friends, family members, coworkers, or romantic partners. But don't assume that having a lot of superficial connections count. They don't. It's nice to have lots of acquaintances, but these less substantial relationships won't feed you the same way deeper connections do. In addition to my friends, I'm fortunate to have plenty of family nearby: my parents, my brother and sister-in-law, and my four nieces. We get together regularly and keep in touch.

Strong relationships can even include pets. Pets can be beloved companions for anyone who needs connection. I have a beloved and adorable greyhound, Ozzie, who greets me in the morning and when I get home, and whom I walk with (not run) at least twice a day. Be sure that no matter who is in your circle of loved ones, you take the time to deeply connect with them. This will improve your daily life and make you so much happier overall.

Create a healthy work/life blend. Too much stress can make you sick, and unfortunately the workplace is a primary source of intense, ongoing stress for many people. That's why it's imperative to play hard in addition to working hard. You need to give yourself permission to blow off steam in a healthy and productive manner (which is one reason why it's so universally rewarding and even relaxing to go for a run or hit the gym after work!).

Make sure you *make* time for relaxation and play. Sometimes people overwork simply because they have no other interests in their life. If you don't have a hobby or set of interests outside of the office, make it your priority to find something to help you unwind. Be adventurous. Try new things. And for goodness' sake, schedule a vacation for yourself once in a while!

Keep this in mind as well: If you work in a job or field that truly causes you an excessive amount of stress or strife, seriously consider finding a profession that allows you to have a better, healthier lifestyle. You get only one life. Make it one you can enjoy.

Foster a spiritual outlet. Many people find healing and restoration by getting in touch with their spiritual side. Being a "spiritual" person doesn't necessarily involve attending religious services or even subscribing to an organized religion at all—although if you wish to identify with a specific religion, go for it!

Even if exploring your spirituality seems like a strange or mysterious concept, don't worry; there are plenty of ways to "test the waters" and see what, if anything, resonates with you. Consider daily practices like meditation or prayer (we'll cover some tips for meditating later in this chapter). These simple rituals can be very powerful heart-healing tools, especially if you're going through a life challenge—health or otherwise. The bottom line: Deepening your spirituality is a powerful way to receive peace, grounding, healing, and strength in an often difficult world.

Break negative thought patterns. "Thinking positive" has become a bit of a cliché, but it is truly important for your overall wellness, including the health of your heart. However, giving up negative thinking is easier said than done for many, many people. As an experiment, count the number of times you think a negative thought in an hour, or even in 10 minutes. You may be surprised by the sheer volume of negative information you're feeding your brain day in and day out. But if you can reverse your negative thinking and replace those pessimistic thoughts with hopeful, positive ones, your life could truly change for the better—and you will certainly have a more pleasant daily existence!

Here are some ways to combat chronic negativity:

- **Use exercise to combat depression or negativity.** I've talked about this already in the exercise section of this book, but regular exercise creates endorphins and makes you feel happier, more accomplished, and in control of your life.

It is a great way to stop a negativity spiral in its tracks. If you are feeling hopeless, get up and go for a walk around the block to "reset" your mood. It often gets you moving in the right direction.

- **Use affirmations.** Whether you are stuck in fear, grief, anger, or any other negative feeling, a simple affirmation can help you break out of the cycle. Affirmations are quiet but powerful messages of comfort that you can say to yourself silently or out loud. Feel free to make up your own affirmation that is particularly meaningful to you, or try one of these. Say it over to yourself several times, and really let the message sink in. It works.

  "In this moment, I am safe and all is well."

  "I consciously release the fear I am feeling."

  "I am surrounded by love, and I *am* love."

- **Start a meditation routine.** Meditation can drastically change your life by keeping you centered and quieting a worried mind. Though it may seem intimidating if you haven't tried it yet, meditation mainly consists of quieting your mind and breathing normally. That's it.

  If meditation is new to you, here's how to begin: Find a quiet space and sit comfortably, either on the floor or in a chair. Close your eyes and try to quiet your mind. Now take a slow, steady inhalation, focusing on your breath. When your lungs are comfortably full, gently exhale. Repeat this process for one minute, and during this time release any thoughts that appear in your mind.

  Congratulations, you've just meditated! Start out meditating for just one minute and gradually work up to five

171

minutes, then ten, and so on. Don't worry too much if you find your mind wandering as you meditate; it's totally normal. Just gently refocus on your breathing when this happens. If it helps, you can count to five as you inhale and exhale, or choose a simple mantra, like *om* or *peace*, to silently repeat with each breath. But again, don't get too hung up on controlling your meditation experience. Paradoxically, meditating is about building discipline *by letting go*. Just try to experience whatever comes in the moment and don't judge yourself.

There are also smartphone apps that can provide you a guided meditation, or help get you started meditating. Headspace and Insight Timer are great sources for beginning a meditation routine.

- **Journal your daily gratitude.** Keep a gratitude journal to remind yourself of the good things in your life. This can give you perspective on bad days when you find yourself falling into a negative mindset. Try to journal a couple of times a week at least. Truly think about your blessings and what your life might be like without them, then write out your reflections.

- **Have a game plan for when you spiral into a "negativity pit."** For those inevitable times when you feel yourself falling into fear, anger, or despair, have a quick plan ready to stop you from spiraling further. Maybe take a five-minute walk or step into a quiet room and breathe deeply for a few minutes until you feel more in control. Or have a quick cuddle with your pet. The point is to be accountable for your mood and outlook by stopping negative beliefs, feelings, and attitudes in their tracks. This helps you reset the pattern and choose a healthier response instead. Over time it will get easier, and you'll automatically default to a more positive outlook.

- **Find a sense of meaning and purpose in your life.** If you haven't already, find something that you care deeply about and incorporate it into your life. This is your purpose; it's what keeps you going through the good times and the bad. Purpose makes everything we've discussed in this book—dietary changes, getting brave enough to try to exercise, and taking charge of your present and future—well worthwhile.

  How do you find your sense of purpose? It can happen various ways. You might align with your purpose by leaving your soul-crushing job to pursue what you really want to do with your life. Or you might find it by adopting a cause that you really believe in and volunteering your time. Or maybe you can find deeper meaning simply by devoting more time to that which brings you pure happiness, such as painting, making music, writing, or singing. Whatever it is, don't ignore your purpose—find a way to incorporate it into your life.

The human experience is full of ups and downs for everyone. It's important to live fully each day, make the most of the good times you have, and work hard to improve on the less-than-perfect aspects of your life that you can change. No matter what's going on with your health, your career, your relationships, or any of your other life circumstances, these guidelines will help ensure that you're not just going through the motions—that you're really living with your *whole heart*.

Whole-hearted living is about tuning into joy, purpose, and wellness so you can face each new day with enthusiasm and vigor. It's a mindset that will help you meet anything that comes your way with a full, rich, and open heart. Just try it and see for yourself. It truly makes a difference.

CONCLUSION

As we approach the end of our journey together, I hope you have a new sense of hope and excitement about a healthier future for yourself. Despite what you may have believed in the past, now you know that heart disease does not have to ruin or even dominate your life. You are armed with the knowledge that small changes can add up to tremendous results. You have learned that the work you put into your health is crucial to maintaining a better quality of life—and that taking back control over your health is much easier than it may seem. My parting advice for you is this:

- Keep it simple.
- Continue making smart food and fitness choices every day.
- Stay in contact with your physician and healthcare team.
- Give yourself credit for small victories.
- Keep trying, even if you make a mistake.
- Treat yourself with kindness—you truly deserve it.

All the best,

Dr. Heather Shenkman

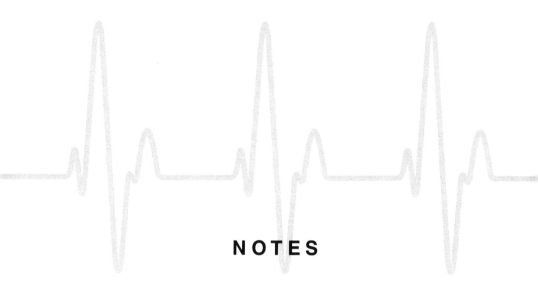

NOTES

Introduction

1. "Heart Disease and Stroke Statistics – At-a-Glance." American Heart Association and American Stroke Association. 2015. https://www.heart.org/idc/groups/ahamah-public/@wcm/@sop/@smd/documents/downloadable/ucm_470704.pdf.

Chapter 2

1. Merai, R., C. Siegel, M. Rakotz, P. Basch, J. Wright, B. Wong, and P. Thorpe. "CDC Grand Rounds: A Public Health Approach to Detect and Control Hypertension." *MMWR Morb Mortal Wkly Rep* 65, no. 45 (November 18, 2016): 1261–4.

2. Mozaffarian, D., E.J. Benjamin, A.S. Go, D.K. Arnett, M.J. Blaha, M. Cushman, S. de Ferranti, et al. "Heart disease and stroke statistics—2015 update: a report from the American

Heart Association." *Circulation* 131, no. 4 (2015): e29-322.

3. Ibid.

4. Ibid.

5. Stamler, J., D. Wentworth, and J.D. Neaton. "Is Relationship Between Serum Cholesterol and Risk of Premature Death From Coronary Heart Disease Continuous and Graded? Findings in 356,222 Primary Screenees of the Multiple Risk Factor Intervention Trial (MRFIT)." *JAMA* 256, no. 20 (1986): 2823-8.

6. "Cholesterol Levels: What You Need to Know." *NIH MedlinePlus*, 2012. Accessed December 21, 2016. https://medlineplus.gov/magazine/issues/summer12/articles/summer-12pg6-7.html.

7. Stone, N.J., J.G. Robinson, A.H. Lichtenstein, C.N. Bairey Merz, C.B. Blum, R.H. Eckel, A.C. Goldberg, et al. "2013 ACC/AHA Guideline on the Treatment of Blood Cholesterol to Reduce Atherosclerotic Cardiovascular Risk in Adults: A Report of the American College of Cardiology/American Heart Association Task Force on Practice Guidelines." *Circulation* 129 (2014): S1-S45.

8. Nissen, S.E., S.J. Nicholls, I. Sipahi, P. Libby, J.S. Raichlen, C.M. Ballantyne, J. Davignon, et al. "Effect of Very High-Intensity Statin Therapy on Regression of Coronary Atherosclerosis: The ASTEROID Trial." *JAMA* 295, no. 13 (2006): 1556-65.

9. Shepherd, J., S.M. Cobbe, I. Ford, C.G. Isles, A.R. Lorimer, P.W. MacFarlane, J.H. McKillop, and C.J. Packard. "Prevention of coronary heart disease with pravastatin in men with hypercholesterolemia. West of Scotland Coronary Prevention

Study Group." *N Engl J Med* 333, no. 20 (November 16, 1995): 1301-8.

10. Scandinavian Simvastatin Survival Study Group. "Randomised trial of cholesterol lowering in 4444 patients with coronary heart disease: the Scandinavian Simvastatin Survival Study (4S)." *Lancet* 344, no. 8934 (November 19, 1994): 1383-9.

Chapter 4

1. Kell, John. "Lean times for the diet industry." *Fortune*, May 22, 2015. Accessed February 28, 2016. http://fortune.com/2015/05/22/lean-times-for-the-diet-industry/.

2. U.S. Department of Health and Human Services. *Women and Smoking: A Report of the Surgeon General.* Rockville, MD: Dept. of Health and Human Services, Centers for Disease Control and Prevention, National Center for Chronic Disease Prevention and Health Promotion, Office on Smoking and Health, 2001.

Chapter 5

1. "American Heart Association Recommendations for Physical Activity in Adults." American Heart Association. July 27, 2016. http://www.heart.org/HEARTORG/HealthyLiving/PhysicalActivity/FitnessBasics/American-Heart-Association-Recommendations-for-Physical-Activity-in-Adults_UCM_307976_Article.jsp#.V7-8RZgrLIU.

Chapter 6

1. Cohen, D.L., L.T. Bloedon, R.L. Rothman, J.T. Farrar, M.L. Galantino, S. Volger, C. Mayor, P.O. Szapary, and R.R. Townsend. "Iyengar Yoga versus Enhanced Usual Care on Blood Pressure in Patients with Prehypertension to Stage I Hypertension: a Randomized Controlled Trial." *Evid Based Complement Alternat Med* 2011 (2011). https://www.ncbi. nlm.nih.gov/pmc/articles/PMC3145370/.

2. "Yoga for anxiety and depression." Harvard Health, April 2009. Accessed January 2, 2017. https://www.health.harvard. edu/mind-and-mood/yoga-for-anxiety-and-depression.

Chapter 8

1. "Modern Animal Farming." Vegan Outreach. Accessed August 30, 2017. https://veganoutreach.org/modernfarms/.

2. "Chickens Used for Food." PETA. Accessed August 30, 2017. https://www.peta.org/issues/animals-used-for-food/facto- ry-farming/chickens/

3. "Modern Animal Farming." Vegan Outreach. Accessed August 30, 2017. https://veganoutreach.org/modernfarms/.

4. Ibid.

5. Wolff, Anita. "The Pros and Cons of Fish Farming" *Ency- clopædia Britannica Advocacy for Animals*, August 4, 2008. Accessed August 9, 2015. http://advocacy.britannica.com/blog/ advocacy/2008/08/the-pros-and-cons-of-fish-farming/

6. Orlich, M.J., P.N. Singh, J. Sabaté, K. Jaceldo-Siegl, J. Fan, S. Knutsen, W.L. Beeson, and G.E. Fraser. "Vegetarian Dietary Patterns and Mortality in Adventist Health Study 2." *JAMA*

Internal Medicine 173, no. 13 (July 8, 2013): 1230-8.

7. Ornish, D., S.E. Brown, J.H. Billings, L.W. Scherwitz, W.T. Armstrong, T.A. Ports, S.M. McLanahan, R.L. Kirkeeide, K.L. Gould, and R.J. Brand. "Can lifestyle changes reverse coronary heart disease?: The Lifestyle Heart Trial." *Lancet* 336, no. 8708 (July 21, 1990): 129-33.

8. Ornish, D., L.W. Scherwitz, J.H. Billings, K.L. Gould, T.A. Merritt, S. Sparler, W.T. Armstrong, et al. "Intensive Lifestyle Changes for Reversal of Coronary Heart Disease." *JAMA* 280, no. 23 (December 16, 1998): 2001-7.

9. Esselstyn, Caldwell B., Jr. *Prevent and Reverse Heart Disease: The Revolutionary, Scientifically Proven, Nutrition-Based Cure.* New York: Avery, 2007.

10. Esselstyn, C. B., Jr., G. Gendy, J. Doyle, M. Golubic, and M.F. Roizen. "A way to reverse CAD?" *J Fam Pract* 63, no. 7 (July 2014): 356-364b.

Chapter 10

1. Centers for Disease Control and Prevention. "State-Specific Trends in Fruit and Vegetable Consumption Among Adults—United States, 2000–2009." *MMWR Morb Mortal Wkly Rep* 59, no. 35 (September 10, 2010): 1125-30. Accessed April 3, 2017. https://www.cdc.gov/mmwr/pdf/wk/mm5935.pdf.

2. Ibid.

3. "Dirty Dozen: EWG's 2017 Shopper's Guide to Pesticides in Produce." EWG. Accessed April 3, 2017. https://www.ewg.org/foodnews/dirty_dozen_list.php.

ABOUT THE AUTHOR

Heather Shenkman, MD, FACC, is an interventional cardiologist in practice in the Los Angeles area. Originally from Detroit, she attended medical school at Albany Medical College and completed her internal medicine residency training at Henry Ford Hospital in Detroit, Michigan. She completed her cardiology fellowship training at the

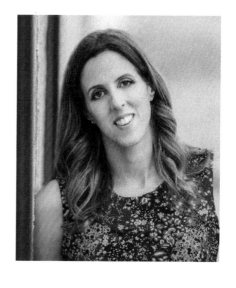

University of Rochester in Rochester, New York, and her interventional cardiology fellowship training at Tufts Medical Center in Boston, Massachusetts.

While she performs complex angioplasties to open up clogged coronary arteries, she prefers to help her patients reduce their risk of heart disease through not only medication, but also a healthy lifestyle, including a plant-based diet and regular exercise.

Dr. Shenkman has followed a plant-based diet since 2005. She is an avid athlete, having completed over 100 events of various distances, from sprint triathlons to Ironman distance triathlons, marathons and ultramarathons, and several 100-mile century cycling events.

Dr. Shenkman is a strong believer in a plant-based diet for heart health, as numerous studies have demonstrated its benefits in the prevention and even reversal of coronary artery disease. A plant-based diet has fueled her athletic success, and she encourages her patients toward this diet for their own health as well.

For more information, please visit www.drheathershenkman.com.

Follow her on Twitter @veganheartdoc.